Praise for *Disease Knows No Politics*

"Elias Zerhouni writes compellingly, and with remarkable modesty, candor, and good humor, about his extraordinary successes as a medical scientist, practitioner, executive, and engineer in academia, government, and industry."—**Harold Varmus**, former director of the National Institutes of Health and Nobel laureate

"From Algeria to the NIH, this memoir spans the American dream."—**Richard Klausner**, former director of the National Cancer Institute and former executive director for global health of the Bill & Melinda Gates Foundation

"From humble beginnings in an Algerian village to his trials and triumphs leading America's biomedical empire, we glean pearls about leadership, integrity, and compassion—virtues Elias Zerhouni exemplifies as few others could. For those interested in medicine, health, and science, *Disease Knows No Politics* is a must-read book." —**Thomas Insel**, former director of the National Institute of Mental Health and author of *Healing: Our Path from Mental Illness to Mental Health*

"*Disease Knows No Politics* is both memoir and manifesto, reminding us of the need to keep partisan politics out of the treatment of disease and the importance of vigilantly protecting the NIH from encroaching ideological forces."—**Jim Greenwood**, former congressman and president emeritus of the Biotechnology Innovation Organization

"I have admired Elias Zerhouni and his insights into individuals and institutions for nearly thirty years. This delightful memoir details how these abilities evolved and enabled him to lead a remarkable life, full of lasting impacts on the many organizations he touched."—**Jeremy Berg**, former editor in chief of the *Science* family of journals and former director of the National Institute of General Medical Sciences

"*Disease Knows No Politics* is, by any definition, a success story. This memoir, written by Elias Zerhouni, provides a roadmap on how to manage whatever circumstances life provides. The guiding theme is to develop basic principles that encourage positive interactions with others for the benefit of all parties involved."—**Phil Frost**, CEO and chairman of OPKO Health

"This memoir reveals the blueprint for leadership and innovation that has served Dr. Elias Zerhouni well through countless triumphs in business, government, medicine, and science."—**Steven Rales**, chair of the board and cofounder of Danaher and Oscar-winning film producer

"Dr. Elias Zerhouni's inspirational journey is a call to action for those who dream of bettering the world and, in doing so, forging a life of adventure and hope."—**Ernesto Bertarelli**, cochair of the Bertarelli Foundation and chair of B-FLEXION

"Zerhouni's vivid memoir of a life devoted to pathbreaking science and its translation directly into the lives of patients and citizens should be read by anyone interested in sound policymaking and audacious leadership for the common good."—**Ronald J. Daniels**, president of Johns Hopkins University and former provost of the University of Pennsylvania

"Dr. Zerhouni is an expert medical scientist, innovator, and entrepreneur whose skills set him apart from others. This memoir illustrates his inspiring life journey with compelling detail. It's a must-read book for all young scientists seeking to make an impact."—**Ed Miller**, former CEO of Johns Hopkins Medicine and former dean of the Johns Hopkins University School of Medicine

"Within fifteen minutes of meeting him, it was clear to me that Dr. Elias Zerhouni was an idea-engine in a vehicle that was driving its chassis into glancing collisions with traditional guardrails. *Disease Knows No Politics* brings readers the life story of a tireless innovator and brave leader."—**Elliot McVeigh**, codirector of the Center for Cardiovascular Biomedical Imaging at UC San Diego

"The melting pot we call America has enabled Dr. Zerhouni's remarkable successes, yet this country has been immeasurably enriched by his pioneering contributions to biomedical research and global health."—**Gary Nabel**, president and CEO of ModeX Therapeutics, chief innovation officer of OPKO Health, and former director of the National Institutes of Health's Vaccine Research Center

"After thirteen years of badgering my longtime friend, Dr. Elias Zerhouni, to bring his unbelievable immigrant story and transformative lessons to the page, he finally has." —**Bruce Holbrook**, president of Bruce Holbrook Consulting, Inc., and recipient of the William & Mary 2022 Alumni Medallion Award

"Braiding themes of scientific discovery and values-driven leadership, this book tells a life story of a true renaissance man."—**Amelia M. Arria, PhD**, professor and associate dean for strategic initiatives at the University of Maryland School of Public Health

"Abraham Lincoln once said, 'Each one of you may have through this free government which we have enjoyed, an open field and a fair chance for your industry, enterprise and intelligence.' Dr. Elias Zerhouni, and his memoir, embody this principle, and it is individuals like him who contribute to making the United States the great nation it is today."—**Mark Devlin**, former president of Computerized Imaging Reference Systems and current president of the phantoms and lasers division at Sun Nuclear

"Zerhouni is a problem solver, a fixer, and a grower—a businessman with an MD. I once told him early in our relationship that he should be running a billion-dollar company. My only regret is that George Bush nabbed him before we had the chance to build the largest radiology company in the country."—**Bob Carfagno**, former CEO of American Radiology Services

DISEASE KNOWS NO POLITICS

former NIH director
DR. ELIAS ZERHOUNI
with EDWARD KRIZ

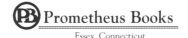
Prometheus Books
Essex, Connecticut

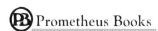

Prometheus Books

An imprint of The Globe Pequot Publishing Group, Inc.
64 South Main Street
Essex, CT 06426
www.globepequot.com

Distributed by NATIONAL BOOK NETWORK

British Library Cataloguing in Publication Information Available

Library of Congress Cataloging-in-Publication Data Available

ISBN 9781493090624 (cloth : alk. paper) | ISBN 9781493090631 (epub)

∞™ The paper used in this publication meets the minimum requirements of American National Standard for Information Sciences—Permanence of Paper for Printed Library Materials, ANSI/NISO Z39.48-1992.

Disclaimer

A memoir is a deeply personal recollection of one's own truth and life. Accordingly, *Disease Knows No Politics* does not claim to provide or possess the ultimate truth regarding any matter, person, or event. We acknowledge the inherent subjectivity of memory, and the stories that follow are told as Dr. Zerhouni remembers them.

Contents

Foreword
An Uncommon Mind

DR. WILLIAM R. BRODY

D
r. Elias Zerhouni has an uncommon mind. He's a once-in-a-generation talent. He thinks on a different plane. Where others see problems, he sees solutions.

Through his memoir, you'll see how his mind works. You'll learn lessons in leadership and life. You'll witness pivotal battles, challenges, and triumphs in politics, medicine, and business.

Elias is a lifelong friend. We've been colleagues, research partners, and entrepreneurs. I've often seen him take A and B to make C, even when A and B seemed unrelated. For example, while at Johns Hopkins Medicine, Elias used magnetic resonance imaging (MRI) to noninvasively put a magnetic tag on the beating heart to detect abnormalities. He took what was known about MRI and what was needed for cardiac imaging and put them together. It was revolutionary.

Elias faced new challenges when, in 2002, President George W. Bush picked him to lead the world's largest public funder of biomedical research and most respected engine of innovation in medicine and health: the National Institutes of Health (NIH). With a budget of more than $23 billion, this colossal research enterprise, critical in our fight against disease, was facing a crisis. Tools of discovery had changed. Disciplines like engineering needed to be further incorporated into the agency. The NIH needed to be restructured to support crucial multidisciplinary research projects.

Past agency directors hadn't succeeded in restructuring it. The NIH was siloed into powerful institutes that opposed certain reforms that might reduce their funds. Change seemed impossible.

Yet Elias cracked the code. Drawing input from the institutes and scientific community, he built a strategic plan for medical research, a road map focusing "on efforts that no single or small group of institutes or centers could or should conduct on its own."[1] To start supporting the initiatives, Elias moved small amounts of money from the institutes and centers into a common fund. He used this relatively small common fund as a pilot experiment on how the NIH could be better run, giving Congress a demonstration of his vision.

To protect and better fulfill the NIH's new strategic plan for medical research, Elias pushed to make the common fund far larger and drawn directly from the government. In 2006, he orchestrated the passing of the NIH Reform Act with the help of key legislators he'd built relationships with, including the late Senator Ted Kennedy. Pivotal, high-risk multidisciplinary projects and the science and young scientists of the future would be enabled. Meanwhile, the new common fund was colossal. For example, it would collectively total almost $1 billion for fiscal years 2007 and 2008.[2] Elias pulled off a remarkable transformation of the NIH, embodying statesman, scientist, and visionary in the process.

As extraordinary as this accomplishment was, it was just one of many for Elias. An Algerian who came to America with just a few hundred dollars in his pocket, he journeyed to the greatest heights of government, medicine, academia, and business. Despite all the success, he remained affable, humble, and self-effacing. His moral compass, empathy, and unflinching leadership never wavered.

The late Albert Szent-Györgyi, who was awarded the Nobel Prize in Physiology or Medicine in 1937, once asserted, "Discovery consists of seeing what everybody has seen and thinking what nobody has thought."[3]

This quote encapsulates who Elias is: one who sees solutions where others see only problems. An uncommon mind.

Introduction

ELIAS ZERHOUNI

"First and foremost, I believe that disease knows no politics."[1]

I spoke these words with conviction during my testimony for the Senate confirmation hearing in 2002 that would usher in my tenure as director of the National Institutes of Health (NIH). For me, these words would be a guiding star as I steered the NIH through stormy political waters, including the embryonic stem cell research debate. As director, I believed the agency's mission was sacred. The NIH needed to be at the service of all Americans regardless of their political preferences, race, sexual orientation, religion, or gender. No disease could be off limits.

Among the many lessons I've included in this memoir, that disease knows no politics is paramount. It refers to how the NIH should function and how our society should manage its staggeringly dysfunctional health care system. To the greatest extent possible, science and public health must be kept separate from partisan politics. Unfortunately, in the present, this fragile modus vivendi has been broken far too often by ill-advised politicians whose narratives, designed to gain or retain power, collide with contradictory scientific evidence. Direct attacks on prominent and respected scientists and government agencies have become worryingly frequent. Likewise, I've also witnessed scientists who have not hesitated to inject their political views into issues they fail to fully comprehend. Despite the changing norms, the NIH and other key government health agencies must be kept above politics, as disease knows none and can affect every one of us regardless of our party affiliation.

Accordingly, this book is for Republicans, Democrats, Independents, and those without party affiliation. It's for scientists and doctors and those without any scientific or medical background. Here, no reader is off limits.

Meanwhile, I provide readers with a counterpunch to lies and conspiracy theories aimed at the NIH and America's scientific community. These falsehoods are damaging, and they breed a distrust that can, in turn, lead patients to abstain from necessary medical care, including vaccines.

Meanwhile, when it comes to medical care, tragically, our health care system has become captive to powerful special interests, supported by, in my view, ill-advised partisan policies that have been promulgated largely by specific members of the U.S. Congress. Patients themselves, the ultimate supposed beneficiaries of our care, have no true place at the table. It's politics and failed policy that are shaping the treatment of disease. When I immigrated to the United States in 1975, I saw its health care system as the best in the world. Regrettably, I no longer believe this to be the case.

By illustrating my life story, including my career in academia, government, and industry, I highlight the negative and positive transformations in U.S. health care and science. I give a sense of the forces at play in and the reality of these institutions and extract lessons applicable to life and work. Accordingly, this book can also serve entrepreneurs, politicians, scientists, doctors, academics, and other professionals looking to improve their lives and those of others.

Finally, in recounting my immigrant journey, starting with its Algerian origins, I want readers to understand that only in America could I have risen so high. I owe much of my success to the greatness of this country and all the rest to my wife and tireless supporter, Nadia. America rewards merit and opens the door for immigrants like me to make lasting contributions that benefit all citizens. I want readers to understand that all I've achieved would not have been possible if America had closed its doors to immigrants of talent. If we want the creative minds, the leaders, the entrepreneurs, and the reformers of tomorrow to come to our shores, America must embrace policies that welcome their arrival.

ALGERIA

I

Childhood and the War

1

O ne morning in 1961, as the war for Algerian liberation raged, there was a knock on the door of my family home. I was 10 years old and living in Pointe Pescade, a seaside suburb of Algiers. Although we were Algerian, my family and I resided amongst a slew of Pied Noirs (translated as "black feet," the name given to European settlers born in Algeria, French citizens whose ancestors had come from countries such as Italy, Spain, Malta, and Germany),[1] many of whom swore allegiance to France and opposed Algerian independence.

My father opened the door and found a frightened Dr. Kollen, the local physician, waiting for him. The Organisation Armée Secrète (OAS), a secret army of French military deserters and Pied Noirs, was carrying out a reign of terror.[2] They were assassinating educated Algerians. Dr. Kollen told my father we were next on the list of families to be killed.

~

Years before this pivotal knock, before the war, on April 12, 1951, I was born in a village in western Algeria, called Nedroma. Local legend claimed the name meant "against Roma," in the spirit of a village that had fiercely resisted all invaders since Roman times. Nedroma was nestled at the feet of Mount Fellaoucene, and in the distance, miles away, one saw the shimmering blue waters of the Mediterranean.

Of the estimated 12,000 inhabitants, most were Muslims (Islam was the religion practiced by most Algerians), and the rest were Jewish. Like many North African cities, Nedroma was influenced by Moorish culture, which was shaped by Muslim and Jewish refugees who arrived during the Middle

Ages after being expelled from Spain. They brought back an extraordinarily rich heritage from Andalucia, with its music, art, cuisine, and science.

Although influenced by Andalucia, my family were indigenous to North Africa, and their Berber origins were embedded in its history. Our ancestral home was in Morocco, and the village my family came from was Moulay Idriss Zerhoun, not far from the haunting, crumbling ruins of the ancient Roman city of Volubilis.

How my ancestors arrived in Nedroma, hundreds of miles away, was a mystery. Documents and memories traced our presence in the village back to 1740. Prior to that, it was possible that our tribe joined the invasion of Spain in the eighth century, only to be expelled back into Algeria when the Spanish Christians reconquered Andalucia.

~

My earliest memory of life—and my only one of Nedroma from those days—was a vivid image of my nine-year-old brother Moustafa riding a bicycle. I was two or perhaps two and a half years old. Soon after, in 1953, we left the village.

My father took our family to Algiers, the capital city. He bought an old house in Pointe Pescade, where he would teach middle school math and physics.

With its lovely beaches, Pointe Pescade was a resort a few miles west of the capital. Our two-floor house was near the beach. My second-earliest memory was inside it. My mother was sitting on the floor, peeling a boiled egg for me. The room was white. The floor had hexagonal red tiles.

As I grew and became more conscious of the world around me, much of it remained beyond my understanding. France had invaded Algeria in 1830 and gone on to settle the country with Europeans at the expense of the indigenous Algerian population.

Pied Noirs made up the majority of Pointe Pescade. Aside from the wealthier residents, most of these Europeans were not ethnically French. Some were Spanish, Italian, or Maltese families who had lived in Algeria since colonial times. Others were Jews who had been there for centuries.

My family was one of only a few Algerian Muslim families in the town. The others resided in poverty in the hills above. Algerians generally worked menial jobs. They were day laborers and servants. In the land of their birth, they were deprived of a better future. At the time, I didn't understand how unjust the situation was or how much worse things were in the countryside. I was just a child being raised by two gifted parents.

~

My father, Mohamed, had a strong, stocky build and a powerful voice. His serious, piercing eyes were set amidst an olive complexion. He was always in good health, and he had a remarkable memory to go along with a sharp, analytical mind. He taught physics and mathematics and was articulate in Arabic and French. His students loved him. He was a magnificent teacher. Although a stern man, like many Algerians, my father also had a sense of humor.

Born in Nedroma in 1914, my father faced early tragedies. His mother died when he was eight. His father was a weaver who went blind and could barely support the family.

As a child, my father grew up in a Nedroma ruled by the French. French occupation had two faces: one of domination, expropriation, and ethnic cleansing and another of bringing "civilization" to indigenous Algerians. French laic and religious educators led efforts to establish schools around Algeria. One such teacher, Mr. Cordell, became a legend in Nedroma, as he established the first Western school in the town. He convinced my grandfather and the elders that my father and the other children would have a better future if they received a Western education.

The elders agreed that Algerian children could attend Mr. Cordell's French school as long as they were not taught religion and continued their traditional Arabic and Koranic education. This meant my father had to attend traditional religious classes from 5:30 to 8:30 in the morning, followed by French schooling until late afternoon. After a quick snack, my father returned to traditional Algerian schooling until the last prayer of the day, which was before bedtime.

My father excelled in his studies. Among other feats, he learned to recite the Koran forward and backward.

He disliked the Koranic teachers, however. They tended to physically punish their pupils in the name of discipline and perfection. My father felt the pedagogy they used was retrograde at best. It encouraged obscurantism, and it was a disservice to the true principles of Islam. He would never allow me or any of my brothers to attend such religious schools.

In contrast, my father enjoyed the methods of his French teachers, who encouraged curiosity and problem-solving. French instructors like Mr. Cordell trained a generation of Algerian students like my father, who then educated the next generation of Algerian leaders.

Unfortunately, the French colonial government did not allow Algerian students to graduate beyond the equivalent of tenth grade. At this time, a few were selected to attend collegiate programs to train them to either teach or otherwise serve the French administration. My father was chosen for the teaching program, yet he resented how European students were given opportunities he was denied.

One of his greatest regrets was never being able to attend university. As a result, he poured all his focus into making sure his seven sons engaged in rigorous education and study en route to pursuing higher degrees. Not much mattered to him beyond our success at school. He spent countless hours coaching us. We had to be first or second in our class. We were not allowed to fail.

~

My mother, Yamna, was beautiful. Her nickname was Houbaya, which meant "the lovely." Like my father, she also wanted her seven sons to receive a strong education.

She had been deprived of one beyond the third grade. The village school for girls had accepted only Europeans or daughters of families that were friendly with French authorities. Despite being a good student, my mother was expelled. To the end of her life, at the age of 92, she mentioned this injustice with tears in her eyes.

My mother educated herself with my father's help. He taught her how to read French. He brought her books to study. She also followed along with our homework. In time, my mother became well-read. She breezed through novels, plays, and other works. She was able to dissect and discuss them with ease.

My mother had an extraordinarily intuitive form of intelligence. She did not follow common wisdom. She had her own way of understanding people and situations. Not surprisingly, she had a strong, independent streak. Never one to conform, she was fearless in the face of adversity.

"Why not try something different?" she'd assert (although it usually had to be her solution).

She was always ready to deflate those who inflated themselves too much. And she had a sharp sense of humor that could leave us all laughing.

Yet my mother also carried a deep sadness over the loss of her first child. During World War II, my sister, Chahida, died of measles. She was only 18 months old. My mother prayed to have another girl. Instead, she had seven boys in a row: Ahmed, Chahid, Moustafa, Boumediene (he would go by Diden), myself, Adnan, and Moulay, in that order.

To remind her of Chahida, my mother required that us boys keep our hair girlishly long and braided until we were old enough to begin schooling. Then our hair was cut. Throughout the rest of her life, my mother kept our severed, braided locks.

〜

In 1956, at the age of five, my long hair and braids were cut, and I began my schooling. My father had me start a year early. In his mind, if I ever had to redo a year, I would be even in age with my classmates. His decision impacted the rest of my life. I would always be the youngest in every class I attended.

My first-grade teacher, Mrs. Torres, was kind and affectionate. She distributed stick-on gold stars for good behavior or improvements in reading or recitation. Most of my classmates were Pied Noirs, and we were taught that our ancestors were the ancient Gauls of France. It was an attempt to erase Algerian history and identity. Yet I did not see myself in the image of the blond kings of Gaul. Except for Pied Noirs whose parents were of French descent, no one else did either.

As first grade continued, so did the war for independence, pitting the French against Algerians of the Front de Libération Nationale (FLN). Trucks filled with French soldiers were a frequent sight. The conflict had begun in 1954. From 1956 to 1957, the Battle of Algiers, in which countless Algerians were tortured and murdered by the French, would erupt close to home and lead to an FLN defeat in the capital.[3]

Wider support for the FLN and their will to fight for Algerian freedom could not be eradicated, however. Among the horrific crimes the French had committed since their invasion in 1830, Algerians would never forget the Sétif and Guelma massacre on May 8, 1945, Victory in Europe Day.[4] Many Algerians had peacefully marched for liberation, brutal conflict had ensued, and, in the aftermath, thousands of Algerians had been murdered.

After this, many Algerians had lost hope of reaching a modus vivendi with the colonizers. It was freedom or death. As for the French, after losing in Vietnam, some were determined to keep Algeria. It was a matter of honor. Also, many French still considered Algeria an intrinsic part of France, destined to be forever French.

I was mostly unconscious of these tensions and would be until the age of eight or nine. Meanwhile, my parents held differing opinions of the war. My father believed the French would eventually recognize equal citizenship rights for Algerians under fair and democratic rules. My mother thought the French would never relinquish their oppressive policies. It was our duty to fight them to the end.

The French themselves held opposing views of the conflict. While the violence against Algerian rebels was welcomed by some Pied Noirs, soldiers drafted from France would object to the inhumane and unjust war. Returning to their country, they shared stories of atrocities committed against Algerians. Many in France began to see the war in a different light than the Pied Noirs.

Additionally, some teachers who had come from France did not support their country's side in the war. Their mission was to uphold equality, fraternity, and freedom. This conflicted with the cruelty that governed French Algeria. These teachers were attentive to the Algerian students, whose only option was to study harder and be better than their domineering and racist Pied Noirs classmates.

∼

Although the war thundered on, I greeted summer with a smile. Summer in the Mediterranean was magic. From June to September, I went to the beach every day, yet only after I had done my chores, part of a rigorous schedule my mother established for her boys. At the beach, I played with friends or went snorkeling and spearfishing along the rocky coasts, catching octopuses and all sorts of fish. The joy of entering clear, turquoise waters was imprinted in my brain, to be the subject of dreams forever after.

I fell in love with the sea. It became an intrinsic part of me. Every morning, I would take in its beauty. I was fascinated with the way that the water's color changed with the weather. Sometimes it was so blue and so flat that there were no waves. When it was like this, we called it a sea of blue oil, or "mer d'huile bleue."

I learned to swim quite early in life, developing an amazing capacity to dive and hold my breath. A problem with my knees made it easier to swim than run, so I naturally chose the former. In the water, I thrived and explored, not unlike Jacques Cousteau, whose documentaries I consumed.

From the morning until late afternoon, I lived amongst the coral reef and its fish. Afterward, I returned to land, starving. Thankfully, my mother always had food put aside for me.

∼

At home, we spoke French and Arabic. While I was in second grade, a new rule forbade students from speaking the latter. One day, an Algerian classmate, Kefous, came to me with a look of mischief. He wanted to play a prank on someone, and he asked me, in Arabic, to help. I responded in

Arabic, not realizing that our teacher, Mrs. Calatayud, was listening. She punished us by striking our fingers with a metal ruler. The blows were heavy and painful. As she hit us, the Pied Noir students cheered her on, hatred in their eyes.

In my class, I was far outnumbered by Pied Noirs. I was also the youngest and not the strongest physically, and I often perceived things differently than others. Not surprisingly, I was bullied. The jabs could be racist.

Yet I found ways to stand up to my adversaries. I was better at swimming than any of them, and I would settle scores by taking them on in the water when they went swimming. This strategy proved successful, as it dissuaded many from picking fights with me. It was my first lesson in understanding the balance of power in hostile relationships. You needed to find your high ground, fight from there, and impose a dissuasive cost on your opponent.

∿

The year 1958 proved to be a turning point in a war that was omnipresent. In France, the Fourth Republic fell, and General Charles de Gaulle became president of the newly formed Fifth Republic.[5] At school, we had to attend a flag-raising ceremony. The French national anthem, "La Marseillaise," was sung. Several Algerian students only pretended to sing it. One of them told me to silently sing the Algerian resistance anthem, "Kassamen," instead. Despite the risk of punishment, I ended up mumbling the anthem with my fellow Algerians, keeping to the tune of "La Marseillaise."

When it came to trying to end the war, Charles de Gaulle used a "stick and carrots" approach. The military campaign was escalated, and reform of socioeconomic conditions and civil administration was overseen.[6] It was too little, too late. Most Algerians no longer believed or trusted that any solution aside from complete independence would work.

∿

At the age of nine, my father sent me to a six-week summer camp in the Pyrenees Mountains of France, where it was safer. Because of the war, I had never spent a summer away from home.

I crossed the shimmering sea on a passenger ship, surrounded by porpoises. I loved it. I arrived in Sète, along with the other Algerian children, and was surprised to not see soldiers. I had grown accustomed to living in a war.

Buses took us into the sharp-peaked Pyrenees. Out here, there was peace. We arrived at a tiny village called Estarvielle, not far from the Spanish border. We were housed in refurbished barns, converted into dormitories, able to fit all 100 of us Algerian children. As we settled in, preparing to go to sleep, no one mentioned the war.

The first weeks were full of discoveries. I experienced mountain life, exploring forests, prairies, and streams. I saw cows and even bears. I was far from the world I knew. We visited nearby towns with beautiful stone buildings and castles bearing scars from a bygone age. I learned to appreciate the true France.

However, after the third or fourth week, I became homesick. My father had signed me up for two consecutive sessions of three weeks. Considering I had never left my family, this was a long time. I missed them—and the sea.

Later, after camp had ended, as I sat on the bus back to Sète, I couldn't wait to see the Mediterranean. At a high turn in the mountains, it appeared, peeking over the horizon. I cried. It was magnificent. My sadness lifted. I was going home.

~

In the Mediterranean, one saw hefty, big-mouthed groupers come in from afar to breed. I was 10 years old, spearfishing with a friend in the waters off Pointe Pescade, when I saw a colossal grouper arrive. It was likely 100 pounds. Speargun in hand, I swam down until I was right in front of the fish.

I cocked my weapon, hesitating. The grouper was so massive that if I speared him, he might drag me deep into the sea and kill me. Yet it wasn't just my survival I was concerned about. As I stared at this giant, magnificent creature, its globular eyes brimming with life, I felt my grip on the gun loosen. Why should I kill it? Why should something so beautiful die?

I lowered my weapon and let the grouper pass on.

~

While I had mastered life in the sea, on land, and in the classroom, there were things I struggled with. One issue was my poor handwriting. My father and brothers had beautiful, calligraphy-like penmanship. I could barely read mine, and I received demerits because of it.

One day, in fifth grade, my class took a math test. I was quite proficient in mathematics, and I swiftly solved each problem. I wrote the answers as neatly as possible. After finishing, I read it all over. I thought my penmanship looked amazing for a change. Proud of my work, I handed in the completed test.

The day arrived when my teacher, Mr. François, finished grading them. He announced that I answered every question correctly, yet because of my poor handwriting, he would impose four penalty points. This put me behind a classmate I was competing with.

I was so hurt, I cried. This was insanity. Understanding something and correctly solving a problem was far more vital than having handwriting that resembled calligraphy.

As I walked home, sulking and distressed, I felt a new determination sweep over me: I would no longer let my poor handwriting stand in my way. Yet how would I overcome this problem? Despite my best efforts, I'd failed to improve my penmanship. I needed to find a different way.

I forced myself to mentally visualize and logically organize whatever was being taught. This lessened the amount of note-taking I did while allowing for more focus and attention on what was being said. By discovering and using an alternative method, I began to synthesize and grasp reality differently. It would prove to be a great strength throughout my life. My physical handicap turned into an intellectual advantage.

The Blue Night 2

Wanting to end an increasingly onerous and unpopular war, de Gaulle moved toward allowing Algerian independence, while Pied Noirs clung to the hope of Algeria remaining French. In 1961, rebellious generals tried to oust de Gaulle. The putsch failed.

The newly born, merciless terrorist organization, the OAS, targeted those in favor of negotiations with the FLN, including French citizens. They also tried to prevent any indigenous intelligentsia from emerging. Algerian doctors, writers, and teachers were assassinated. My father was scared.

Daily bombings destroyed government buildings, hotels, and schools. The explosions culminated in a terrifying evening of destruction in which an estimated 120 bombs were planted in Algiers. It came to be known as the "Blue Night."

On this night, the city shook. My family and I hid under our beds, hearts pounding as the explosions came closer and closer, until the post office 200 meters away was destroyed. Would we be next?

Slowly, the explosions faded into the west side of town. We were alive, for now.

～

School was often closed, forcing us to stay home. My father let us leave only for essential errands. My brothers and I taught ourselves the subjects we would've studied in class. As a result, I developed an independent approach to learning that served me well throughout my life.

Yet my studies could not distract me from the world beyond my home, which was crumbling into unspeakable violence. The OAS was killing every Algerian in sight. Women who worked as cooks and handmaids were shot on their way to work.

My two oldest brothers, Ahmed and Chahid (then 20 and 19 years old, respectively), had gone away for boarding school. One night, while they ate in the cafeteria, an OAS commando entered and opened fire, killing a few students. My brothers escaped and eventually arrived at our home. They stayed rather than returning to their school.

Soon after, a morning came that changed the course of our lives. A knock from our local physician, Dr. Kollen, brought my father to the door, and we discovered we were next on the list of Algerian families to be murdered.

"You've got to leave." Dr. Kollen begged, "Please, please, please, Mr. Zerhouni. Please leave!"

Dr. Kollen was French. He was a kind man who gave us immunizations and kept us well. While he wasn't part of the OAS, other neighbors were. One of them had told him we were on the list.

My father, then acting principal of the school, couldn't believe the parents of the children he cared for could kill us. Dr. Kollen told him the assassination squad wasn't coming from our neighborhood. They would arrive from far away and not know or care about who we were.

As the news sunk in, my father decided to act. We needed to leave immediately. There was a problem, however. My mother and my brothers, Diden and Moulay (the latter was just a baby), were visiting our ancestral village to attend my maternal grandmother's funeral. They were to return in the coming days, unaware of the danger. My father decided he would wait for them, while the rest of us (Ahmed, Chahid, Moustafa, Adnan, and myself) would journey to Nedroma, which was around 350 miles away. Once my mother and other brothers arrived in Pointe Pescade, they and my father would depart.

My father gave money and instructions to Ahmed and Chahid. We were to go by train and bus. We were forbidden from stopping in large cities. That's where the OAS was strong.

The next morning, we took a taxi to the train station. It was driven by Mr. Rosello, a Pied Noir who respected my father. We would one day learn that Mr. Rosello was part of the OAS. We believed he was the one who informed Dr. Kollen we were next on the list.

During the ride to the train station, I wasn't frightened about what was happening. I was 10 years old, and in my mind, we were having an adventure. Although it was dangerous, we were going to survive.

I had my older brothers with me. Who could beat us? And my father was going to be fine. He was so strong and smart. Who could possibly harm him?

Mr. Rosello dropped us at the train station. We entered and ran into my mother, holding my baby brother, Moulay, in her arms, with Diden (who was 12) by her side. My father told us that if we ran into them, we were to instruct them to come with us. We relayed his orders. My mother refused. She wouldn't leave without her husband.

"Go ahead without us. I'll go get him, and then we'll come," she insisted.

We pleaded for her to reconsider, but to no avail. My mother left, taking Moulay and Diden with her.

We took a train destined for Oran, a large coastal city in the northwest, around 260 miles from Algiers. We stopped for the night in a village outside Oran, called Misserghin. OAS commandos had infiltrated the community. Thankfully, one of my father's friends and former colleagues, who was French, looked after us. We spent the night in a horse stable and woke up early the next morning. We traveled by train to Tlemcen and then by bus to Nedroma.

The contrast between Nedroma and Algiers was jarring. I had left the dangerous, urban, heterogeneous world of the city for the relative safety of this homogeneous, rural village. I saw no Pied Noirs speaking French. Only Algerian Muslims and Jews conversing in Arabic.

Horses and donkeys clopped through the marketplace. My nostrils smelled wool being worked to make carpets, part of an economy of arts and crafts. Andalusian music filled the air. I had traveled back to the fifteenth century. Walking the narrow streets, my mouth watered from the scent of delicious Moorish dishes.

Nedroma did have touches of the modern world. It had a post office, electricity, and telephones. The latter were owned only by the wealthy and the French administrators.

Staying at our grandparents' home, my brothers and I were well received. First cousins, second cousins, third cousins, aunts, uncles—all warmly welcomed us. I was able to get to know them.

Not all of them were from the village. Some had also escaped the cities like us. And our family was not the only one in the middle of a reunion. Other refugees were arriving, met with the embrace of their relatives.

Outside this oasis, the reign of terror raged in the cities. We had no way of communicating with my parents, Diden, and Moulay. We didn't know if they were alive. My older brothers, who fully understood what was going on, were worried sick.

One day, a villager ran up to us, bringing wonderful news. Our parents had arrived. They were at the bus station with Diden, Moulay, and our faithful dog, Znouka. On seeing them, I cried.

My parents had hid in our home for a few weeks, giving the impression everyone was gone. Neighbors surreptitiously delivered bread and other necessities until my mother, father, and brothers escaped with the help of the taxi driver, Mr. Rosello, who, apparently, had told the assassination squad commander that our entire family had left town.

～

In Nedroma, my father was asked to take over the school, as many of the French staff were gone. He agreed, under the condition we could live in the apartment of the French principal who had left.

My father reopened the school, and under his care, an institution that had been falling apart was put back together. The village was grateful. Classes started, and my education continued. These were happy days, where I forged lasting friendships and spent time with family.

I adapted to life in Nedroma. The smells, sounds, and sights of the village became familiar. I realized my education and upbringing in Pointe Pescade had left me in the dark about some of my roots. For example, I had a granduncle who was a musician and a poet. His poems were sung in Nedroma, and the local conservatory, el Mossilia, performed his works. I was touched that my family had helped shape the unique Moorish–Andalusian culture of the village.

I also learned that Nedroma had a somewhat democratic government run by elders that maintained law and order with a transparency that French rule lacked. In addition to this democracy, landownership was fundamental to the structure of the village.

My mother explained, "We own lands in the mountains, in the valley, where every year we get almonds. We get the fruits of the production of these lands as our share, which is divided by the inheritance rules amongst myself, my sisters, my brothers."

When someone died, they could also give their land to the community. These land grants were managed by the village council to serve communal needs and take care of the poor.

Many years before my birth, under French rule, this system was violated. The communal lands were taken and divided up amongst Pied Noirs settlers. Additionally, one of the Algerian managers of the non-communal lands owned by my mother's family decided to run them for himself, keeping the spoils. The French helped him.

Meanwhile, my maternal grandfather died at age 49 of what seemed to be a heart attack, leaving my grandmother to raise her eight children (including my mother) alone. Since the Algerian land manager would no longer pay what was owed to my grandmother's family and because the communal land was controlled by Pied Noirs settlers, there was nothing to stop my grandmother and her children from descending into poverty. My mother never forgot the hunger of those years.

In time, the Algerian manager had a severe stroke. His children and advisers told him that he was being punished by God for having sinned against a widow with children and no means. The only way he could be free of his punishment was if he begged the widow's forgiveness. They put the man in a horse carrier and took him to my grandmother's home, bearing gifts.

Barely able to speak, he said, "Please . . . forgive me."

"I've suffered. My children have gone hungry," my grandmother responded, a quiet rage in her eyes. "What you've done is not forgivable by me. You can only be forgiven by God."

One of her sons, Djillali, joined the fight for Algerian liberation, fueled by the pain of his childhood. As an uncle, Djillali would play an invaluable role in my life. While working as a doctor in France, he joined the FLN, which desperately needed physicians. My uncle was sent to a region near the center of Algeria. He ran an FLN war hospital in caves underneath the mountains.

When the French attacked, my uncle was badly wounded. The FLN tried to sneak him out of the country on the back of a donkey through the desert. He and his guide became lost. To survive, my uncle had to drink his own urine. He almost died. By chance, he was found by an FLN unit heading to Morocco. In Morocco, he was taken in by the Swedish Red Cross.

My uncle had a limp for the rest of his life. He would try to hide it, walking in a way that looked somewhat elegant. Forever carrying a reminder of the war.

With the war nearing its end, a free Algeria was on the horizon. My classmates and I were told we would be the future. We needed to excel in our studies.

"Your country is going to need you," my father said to us.

Thousands of Algerian students had been killed. When the war ended, there would be few alive with a university education. Nedroma was unified in its effort to prepare the next generation to fill this void.

Although there may have been unity on some issues, Algerians had divisions that ran deep—divisions I became more aware of. Age-old separation existed between those in the mountains and those in the villages and cities. It was a love–hate relationship.

The people in the mountains were Berbers who stuck to their ancient roots and culture. The people in the villages and cities tended to be Berbers also, yet they were more Moorish in culture. Many in the mountains saw them as invaders who had taken over the country and sold it to the French, collaborating with the colonizers.

When it came to the war, the people of the mountains had borne the brunt of it. In 1962, I visited the mountain where my mother's adopted half sister, Kheira, lived. She spoke a Berber language. Outside her home, Kheira had a garden. Her son, Hocine, who was my age, took me into it.

"I want to show you something. But you can't tell anybody," he said, voice hushed.

He revealed a large cave where his family hid their valuables and food and escaped raids. They lived in constant fear of both the French and the FLN. The latter insisted on having their support.

The cave was big enough for Hocine's entire family to hide in it. When the French would come, the FLN could hide there as well. It was part of a tunnel system. Not far from it, I saw the tombs of freedom fighters.

~

On March 18, 1962, the French and FLN agreed to a ceasefire. FLN troops came down from the mountains and entered the villages and cities. Other FLN soldiers and refugees arrived from Morocco. Meanwhile, the French army progressively left.

With the arrival of the FLN in Nedroma, lambs were sacrificed so that welcome meals could be prepared. It was a triumphant moment. I saw and felt joy.

Yet there was also rage. Wounds inflicted by the French still bled. Many wanted revenge. Algerians who collaborated with the French tried to flee the country. Some were killed before they could. Pied Noirs took part in a mass exodus, with hundreds of thousands leaving Algeria. Many abandoned the Algerians who had helped them.

In a country starving for vengeance, my family had connections to both the freedom fighters who had won the war and the French. A deceased granduncle had received the Legion of Honour. He helped provide supplies to the French army in World War I.

His actions were honorable, yet he died with a reputation of having worked with the French. It was a mark on the Zerhouni family in Nedroma. It would be one of the reasons why my father eventually had us return to Pointe Pescade. He did not want to remain involved in the emerging, intense politics of revenge.

One day, my father didn't return home from the school. An FLN commander had rounded up all educated Algerians, including him. The commander believed they had all collaborated with the French, even though many had left the cities to escape atrocities. The commander brought them to a farm and roughed them up. For 48 hours, we didn't know what was happening to my father. We didn't know if he was alive.

A cousin in the FLN tried to convince the commander to free my father. The commander wouldn't budge. Ultimately, my father's connection to FLN leader Ahmed Ben Bella (who would become the first president of Algeria) saved him. The two knew each other. My father and the others were freed. When my father returned home, he was shaken.

"We're going to go from one dictatorial regime to another," he mourned.

On July 1, a referendum was held for independence, and an overwhelming majority of Algerians voted for freedom.[1] Algeria had finally been liberated.

In Nedroma, there were celebrations. The women let out their traditional cry of joy, the "yoo-yoo." It felt unbelievable to go from French domination to this frenzy of joy and hope. I thought the future would be wonderful.

The elders were not as excited. My father was also skeptical that political unity would remain. In time, his doubts would come true.

Independence and Teenage Years 3

The war had turned Algerians against each other. Independence would as well. Centuries of differences could not be undone. There were those who were French educated. There were those who were educated in Arabic. There were Berbers of the mountains who believed they were the original inhabitants; everyone else was an invader.

During the summer following independence, Algeria fell into civil war, though, soon enough, compromises were made, and a government was agreed to. Ben Bella became prime minister and, later, president of a one-party, FLN-dominated government.

In October, my family and I left Nedroma. The sun was setting when we finally arrived at our home in Pointe Pescade. The house had been ransacked. Most of our stuff was missing. My mother was in tears. Yet at least the OAS was gone. Peace had returned.

The next morning, I stepped into an unfamiliar world. On the streets, I didn't see the usual activity or the people I remembered. I visited the home of a French friend, Jean Fontaine, knocking on the door. An Algerian man whom I'd never seen before opened it.

"What do you want?" he asked.

"Is Jean here?"

"Jean?"

"The boy who lives here."

"There's no Jean here. Get lost."

Next, I went to visit a Jewish friend, David Demri. We had played together many times. He was also gone. And on and on it went. All the buildings were there, yet none of the people I knew were in them. Most of my childhood friends had disappeared.

As I walked the streets, I saw homes occupied by Algerians from the mountains. They had taken the houses over, left empty after the Pied Noir evacuation. I was grateful no one had taken ours.

Yet I was also disoriented. The culture of Pointe Pescade had transformed overnight. My childhood environment was gone. I would have to adapt. I would need to build a new life yet again.

~

Algeria's identity was much in question. It was a heterogeneous nation, influenced by French culture, with a divided population of Berbers. Some spoke a Berber language and stuck to their roots. Others were culturally Arabic and influenced by Islamic values. Amidst a wave of Arab nationalism, Ben Bella aligned with Egyptian president Abdel Nasser; Algeria needed to separate its identity from the French and develop a new one based on Arabic culture.

In terms of the educational system, some felt the future was in going back to Algeria's Arabic roots. Others asserted that a European-style, modern education, including science and technology, was essential. There were also Algerians who believed the future was a synthesis of both.

In this uncertain climate, my father returned to teaching. I returned to class. Before the war, my school's student body had been made up mostly of Pied Noirs. Now, as I entered the doors of Lycee Emir Abdelkader (renamed in honor of a legendary Algerian resistance leader of the nineteenth century), I saw only Algerian students, many having come from rural areas and cities across the country.

Many Algerian teachers and intellectuals had been killed during the war, by both the French and the FLN, leaving schools shorthanded. To help, the French government agreed to keep a cadre of its teachers in Algeria. These teachers were different from the past Pied Noir ones I'd had. They wanted Algerian boys and girls to get the best of both a French and an Arabic education, an opportunity our parents never had.

Seventh grade brought forth a wealth of knowledge. Among other things, I was taught French and French history as well as Arabic and Arabic history. Algeria lacked the teachers needed to educate all of us in Arabic, so Abdel Nasser had sent many from Egypt. Unbeknownst to most Algerians, some of these teachers were said to be imprisoned members of the radical Muslim Brotherhood, which Nasser wanted to get rid of.

"You're ignorant animals," one of these dogmatic, Egyptian teachers told me and my class.

To him, we were primitive and miseducated and contaminated by French culture, and we would not recover our identity until we reconnected with our Arabic roots and language. This teacher's style of pedagogy wasn't engaging, and he knew little beyond the alphabet and key sentences and Koranic sayings. We didn't respect his ignorance and dogmatism.

During my primary school years, when the French had still reigned, I was forbidden from speaking Arabic. Now this Egyptian teacher imposed the opposite rule: we were not allowed to speak French in class. He also didn't let us use our local language, which was Arabic laced with Spanish and French. Anyone who uttered it was punished. He wanted us to speak classical Arabic, which would be like speaking Latin rather than modern French.

We went along with the teacher's rules, participating in the class while understanding that what he taught wasn't the future. The future was in technology. It was in science.

Many didn't like the Arabization strategy. Yet it eventually became dominant, destroying modern education in Algeria. Thankfully, while I was at Lycee Emir Abdelkader, its impact was not as significant. My ignorant Egyptian teacher was an exception, not the rule. The Algerian teachers who educated us in Arabic were completely different. They wanted us to get the best of both an Arabic and a French education.

In terms of my education, I did well in the hard sciences. I loved math and physics, and a student's ability determined the level of each they took. This extended to other subjects as well. There was not just one seventh grade. There were several.

The school sub-characterized the different groups. I was in the one with a scientific emphasis, learning alongside talented classmates.

It was easy to make friends. The tall, blue-eyed Walkhereddine (his mother a German, his father Algerian police) and the friendly Boutouchent were some I wouldn't forget. I connected with my new friends around the notion of being good at what we did in school and working hard. There was a culture of achievement. One-minded competition toward excellence. Having a peer group like this was invaluable. In life, the friends you keep shape your destiny.

My classmate Hachemi, who would become a lifelong friend, was strong in mathematics, just like I was. We bonded over this. We challenged each other. Although he was competitive, Hachemi was also kind. He was a pleasant, charismatic super-connector who brought me into his diverse circle of friends from many different regions of the country. Hachemi himself was from a village in the east.

We shared a dislike of our physical education class (I couldn't run well, as I didn't have good knees), and one day, I proposed that we find a way to get out of it. Hachemi nodded in agreement.

Physical education was right after lunch. Hachemi and I cut our mealtime short and arrived at class before everyone else. Lycee Emir Abdelkader had a basketball court, with a wall separating it from the outside world. We entered the court and scaled the wall, which was about nine feet tall, escaping into the city.

We had plenty of fun. We chased girls. We went to the movies. There was a movie theater called Cinematheque that showed classics for cheap prices. Some were French movies, including the work of director Marcel Carné, and the film trilogy *Marius*, *Fanny*, and *César*, born from famed author Marcel Pagnol. Others were dubbed American movies, such as *Spartacus*.

Over time, we skipped out on physical education again and again, enjoying our trips into the city. Yet one day, we climbed the wall and were shocked to find the principal on the other side. We were caught. It was the end of our excursions, and Hachemi and I had a new reputation. We were kids who needed to be watched.

∼

Lycee Emir Abdelkader was, in many ways, a magnet school, ranked among the best. Yet the curriculum had holes. We lacked the teachers for certain subjects. For example, I never had geology, and for biology, my education was spotty. These educational gaps were a problem.

Students took national exams. If a student's curriculum was full of holes, they would fail these tests. I needed to find a way to fill the gaps in my education.

Working together, my friends and I found the books we needed and educated each other. Given that Algeria was a poor country, there were times when we couldn't obtain the necessary texts, so we went to the cultural centers of the foreign embassies. I would succeed in passing the national exams, though there were gaps in my education that I was never able to fill.

This wasn't the first time I'd relied on self-education. During the war, there were plenty of days when I couldn't go to school. I learned how to teach myself and solve problems on my own. These are essential skills.

∼

My father raised me in a home of math and science. It was an invaluable gift. Yet as much as I appreciated my father's help, I actively avoided having him as a teacher at school.

In eighth grade, when Hachemi and I saw the list of subjects we were going to take, we realized that my father was one of our assigned teachers. I wasn't happy.

I looked at Hachemi, my face pale. "I don't want to be a student in my father's class. I mean, no way. No. Way. Hachemi, I can't do that."

To be the teacher's son in a class was a lose-lose situation. If I did well, everyone would think it was because my father was the teacher. If I didn't do well, everyone would think I was a complete idiot.

"We need to figure a way out of this, Hachemi," I insisted.

Hachemi came up with an idea. The only eighth-grade group my father didn't teach a subject for was the challenging, "super nerd" one. Nobody wanted to be in it. Subjects included Latin, Greek, and a second foreign language. If we switched into it, we could avoid my father.

Typically, when a kid was assigned to that group, they pleaded to get out of it. We did the opposite. We went to the administrator who handled the group assignments and convinced him to switch us into it.

There were fewer kids in our new eighth-grade group than in the more popular, easier ones. The teachers were exceptional and, at times, unorthodox. They favored intellectual stimulation over excessive discipline and rote learning. I had taken a risk and joined a smaller, more elite set of students to escape my father, and in doing so, I unwittingly upgraded my education, impacting the rest of my life.

Soon enough, I made another crucial decision that unintentionally bettered my future. When it came time to choose a foreign language, I entered the sign-up rooms and looked around. For English, the line to enroll was 200 students deep. For Russian, it was 70 students. I saw 50 kids waiting in line for Spanish. The line for German, however, had only nine students. My friend Walkhereddine was one.

I hated waiting in long lines, so I joined him. I signed up for German. It proved to be a fantastic decision. The teacher, Mr. Chabot, was wonderful, and the class was small. I enjoyed learning the language and ended up winning the national prize for German. As part of it, I was sent to Germany for a month. All because I chose the shorter line.

～

In ninth grade, there was an Algerian mathematics teacher, Mr. Tsuria, with a prosthetic eye who taught me a lesson I never forgot. He was a veteran of the war and a genius, with a hippie-like appearance.

He taught by posting problems as case studies and then asking questions. Hachemi and I worked together to come up with answers. We often succeeded. Noting this, Mr. Tsuria looked for a way to challenge us.

The day before winter vacation, he came to class with a problem he wanted all of us to try to solve over break. Whoever did would be rewarded.

Confident and cocky, Hachemi and I got to work. We met often to discuss our progress, which, unfortunately, was nonexistent. No matter how hard we tried, we couldn't find the solution. Day after day, we toiled, vacation drawing closer to an end. Finally, we returned from break, still without an answer.

We entered class. No one else had figured it out either. Our teacher smiled, amused. He revealed that the problem was Fermat's Last Theorem. In hundreds of years, it had never been solved.

I was furious. My teacher had ruined my vacation. However, in looking back on those days, I would come to understand their value. An impossible problem was exactly what we'd needed. Attacking one led to failure, which led to growth. Impossible problems were also an opportunity to make a unique contribution—to do what no one else had done before.

~

During his reign, President Ben Bella enlarged his powers and ruled with instability, repression, and demagogy.[1] In 1965, military leader Houari Boumediene overthrew Ben Bella. Boumediene's austere authoritarianism was aided by the Sécurité Militaire, a political police force.[2]

With a new leader in charge of Algeria, my journey at Lycee Emir Abdelkader continued. I was in tenth grade. I now attended class with both boys and girls.

While my academic education mattered to my parents, they stressed the importance of other activities, such as learning piano at the conservatory. My brother, Diden, came with me, as he was learning to play the trombone.

Another activity I engaged in was competitive swimming. I was terrible at sports on land, yet I could swim well. At the age of 16, I followed a teacher's advice and joined a local swim club.

It was a small team that convened two evenings a week at a pool in the center of Algiers, seven miles or so from Pointe Pescade. After practice, the coach kindly drove us all home in his tiny car. The only girl on the team sat up front. Her name was Nadia Azza. She was 17. One day, I would marry her.

Nadia was born in Sidi Bel Abbès, a city not far from Nedroma. She was the second of four sisters. Her parents met at a swimming pool in Toulouse, France, during World War II. At the time, her French mother had been an exceptional swimmer, and her Algerian father had been a professional soccer player and was also pursuing a law degree. Now her father was a prominent lawyer in Algiers who saw how women were mistreated in society. He made sure all his daughters, Nadia included, received an education to give them more control over their future.

During the war, Nadia had felt the brunt of it. The French Foreign Legion had been based in Sidi Bel Abbès. To escape danger, Nadia and her family had moved to France from 1959 until 1963. Like other Algerians of our generation, Nadia had her life upended by the war.

Now Nadia lived in the center of Algiers, so when our swimming coach drove us all home, he dropped her off first. The first time Nadia and I ever interacted was when she was getting out of the car. I was supposed to take her seat in the front. Before I could, she accidentally shut the door. I was annoyed. She was embarrassed.

As time went on, even though we were both quite shy and our conversations were limited, we got to know each other better. Nadia was soft-spoken, articulate, wise, intelligent, and beautiful. Later in our lives, we would fall in love. For now, we remained acquaintances.

Meanwhile, in the pool, I trained hard. The more I practiced, the more I improved. Around the age of 18, I made it onto the national team.

Competitive swimming was a tremendous character builder. It gave me resilience. I practiced setting goals and committing myself to achieving them. Through this extracurricular activity, I gained essential skills. It was a lesson in the value of athletics and the way in which participating in one activity could help an individual develop the mental skills necessary for success in another.

I would ultimately give swimming up when I arrived at university, yet I'd never completely abandon it. I'd continue to do it throughout my life. The same would be true for playing music. Years later, my son, Will, would recall how I often played the Moorish lute during his childhood (it remains one of my favorite instruments).

With the arrival of twelfth grade, I was in my final high school year. My classroom was where Albert Camus, the Nobel Prize–winning French author, had studied.

Meanwhile, I wanted to become a mathematician or a scientist. I also loved physics and was fascinated by Einstein's work. It was a world I could see myself going into. Yet I was also pragmatic, and part of me wanted to become an engineer. A builder of buildings and bridges in a country that greatly needed modern infrastructures.

My parents encouraged this latter dream. Algeria needed help, and I could contribute. I had always been a tinkerer, building prototypes of things. When I was a toddler, my mother said I would disappear at times. She would find me in the garage working on dissembling a large clock.

"I would find you with all the scattered parts," she said. "Of all the kids, you acted the most like an engineer."

Meanwhile, I was thinking about one day building an enterprise. Maybe in construction or something else. My future had possibilities, and in the late spring of 1968, I graduated from Lycee Emir Abdelkader. With my mind swimming with the dreams of days to come, I had no idea of how much my life's trajectory would evolve and be dictated by unforeseen events.

The University of Algiers   4

I t was 1971, and I was attending the University of Algiers. I was active in student politics, questioning the way Algeria was being run under the rule of Houari Boumediene. Although I was criticizing the government, I didn't feel in danger. My dissent hadn't crossed the line.

One day, much to my shock, I was picked up by the Sécurité Militaire. They accused me of printing communist propaganda. It was a serious crime of which I was innocent. Yet as my interrogation progressed and I tried to talk myself out of the situation, I found the officers unconvinced. In their eyes, I was guilty.

∼

Years before, during the summer of 1968, my first paid job was in a quality control lab for public works. The lab examined the quality of cement, concrete, and steel rods used in construction. Every project needed to fulfill specifications and building codes.

Builders allowed us to examine samples of what they were using. As an assistant in the testing lab, I tested these samples, determining whether they were up to code. For example, we had a compression machine that measured the force at which the concrete samples broke. Similarly, for steel rods, we had a machine that pulled them apart until they cracked.

Among other tasks, I analyzed the components of concrete before they had been fused by water. I used a granulometric analysis, which consisted of passing the mixture through a series of sieves, separating its components. Stones stayed at the top, with pebbles below them and sand below the pebbles. The image of these separated components would stay with me and serve as part of a key metaphor for prioritization that I used later in my life.

One day at work, I came across an unsolved problem. At a construction site, every time they built a wall, it collapsed. Not surprisingly, their concrete samples kept failing our testing. It was driving the developer crazy.

"I'm putting in the right amount of cement," the developer insisted. "I'm putting in the 26 percent, and it's failing."

He was telling the truth. He begged our lab to help him solve the problem.

I did some research. The construction project obtained the rocks for their concrete mixture from a dry riverbed. I analyzed these rocks in the lab. I observed a fine powder, made of organic material, coating all of them. This powder prevented the cement from fusing with the rocks. It was the reason the concrete was failing.

I proposed that the powder be washed from the rocks prior to mixing to allow adherence to the cement. It worked. This was the first research project—and discovery—of my career.

~

I would work in the lab only for several months. I then left to attend the University of Algiers, beginning in the fall of 1968. I moved out of my parents' house and began my classes. I initially pursued a high degree in mathematics and physics.

I hated it. My classmates were dull. The teachers weren't great. When it came to our lessons, they taught us the "what" but not the "why" behind it. Throughout my life, my desire to know the "why" behind things would be an asset, helping me to understand them at a more fundamental level.

As I struggled to enjoy my studies, my brother, Diden, who liked his premed classes, suggested I switch into the program. In the world of medicine, I saw that one could play an active role in helping others. I also had friends in the program, and the women were beautiful. Nadia most of all.

My uncle, Djillali, who was a physician, encouraged me to enter premed. In Sweden, Djillali had studied at the esteemed Lund University, specializing in radiology. Now he wanted me to also pursue a future in medicine. Yet my mother and father were against it. They didn't respect the medical profession.

My father thought it wasn't an intellectually challenging pursuit. To him, medicine was merely learning by rote. A doctor memorized what they needed to know, and then they prescribed drugs in their office.

Thankfully, my uncle convinced my father the profession had changed, and I switched over to premed. I enjoyed my new educational track.

Premed was just the beginning of a larger, seven-year medical curriculum that ended with an internship.

My first two years were enjoyable. I learned the basics, such as biochemistry, biophysics, physiology, and histology. During this period, the dean of the medical school, Dr. Abdelmoumene, reformed the study curriculum so it closely paralleled the one in the United States. He had trained in the United States, including a significant stretch at the NIH. He wanted to revolutionize the study of medicine in Algeria. He did just that.

Despite these positive changes, there was an ongoing problem. In merely filling our heads with facts and formulas, we weren't pursuing the "why" behind the "what." It was similar to my experience in the math and physics program. If I asked questions aimed at discovering the "why," the teachers wouldn't answer them.

"Listen, son," one said. "I've got hundreds of students here. I can't take the time."

I also hated taking notes. It was torture because of my poor penmanship, and, unfortunately, students had to write down every word.

~

Outside the classroom, I became involved in student politics. Friends of mine participated as well. We questioned the way the socialist government was run under President Boumediene. We wanted Algeria to move away from authoritarianism.

We tried to win student elections by opposing the FLN presence within the university. We had general assemblies. We gave speeches. I loved it. It was my first taste of politics.

After taking power in the 1960s, Boumediene had emphasized an Islamic and Algerian brand of socialism.[1] The head of the FLN party, Kaïd Ahmed, was against socialism, though not overtly.

Ahmed once visited the University of Algiers and spoke to students. He was candid, sociable, down to earth, and a showman. People liked him, and he loved talking to us.

"I don't know why you students want to break from the FLN and go with the communists," he stated, setting up a joke. "I mean, I read Karl Marx. I read the entire book. I didn't understand a thing. It made no sense."

There was laughter in the audience. My friend, Walkhereddine, who I'd known since high school, was seated next to me. He wasn't amused by the joke. Unbeknownst to me, he had become a communist.

"You probably didn't understand a thing because there were no pictures," Walkhereddine jabbed back.

The room went silent. My face went pale. I couldn't believe Walkhereddine had said that. I thought the Sécurité Militaire was going to drag us away. To my surprise, Kaïd Ahmed laughed. He wasn't angry.

"You know, son, you're right," he responded with a grin. "There were no pictures because Karl Marx's book made no sense, so he couldn't come up with any pictures to illustrate it."

Again, the audience laughed. Algerians loved humor. It was part of their culture. They liked to make jokes and draw funny cartoons.

I breathed easier. The fact that Walkhereddine and I weren't punished reflected the brotherly atmosphere that existed in Algeria at the time. It wasn't oppressive like in the Soviet Union. Even still, a few months later, the head of the FLN was fired for opposing some of Boumediene's socialist policies.

Algeria had a place in the worldwide socialist movement. Prominent figures such as Fidel Castro and Che Guevara visited the country. At one point, the latter lived near Pointe Pescade. My brothers met him. Che Guevara would go to a local bar and play cards. Algeria was, in a way, a revolutionary place. Leaders from the Black Panther Party were some of the others who visited, Eldridge Cleaver among them, who I saw a few times.

～

As my involvement in student politics progressed, in my studies, my frustration with the rote learning and tedious note-taking continued. Despite these grievances, an experience volunteering in the Algerian countryside would reinforce my commitment to medicine.

I journeyed to a mountainous region in the east of the country to help convince Algerians to buy into Boumediene's socialist agrarian reform. Large farms would have their lands separated. Peasants would work in government-run cooperatives. I had been critical of the FLN in student politics, yet I felt that Algeria needed to modernize its agriculture. This reform seemed like a way to help do that.

To my surprise, the peasants resisted.

"How would you feel if I took the land of your forefathers?" one of them asked me. "If I went to your village and took the land from your family, how would you feel? You'd feel like a new colonizer had arrived, right?"

The government was expropriating the property of wealthy Algerian families who had owned their land for hundreds of years. This peasant didn't have any land, yet he was adamant about not going along with the initiative. To him, it was dishonorable. This peasant—and others—feared God's punishment if they took the land. Additionally, peasants didn't want to work on cooperative farms where the FLN party would run their life. Not surprisingly, the agrarian reform would fail.

During my time in the countryside, I also worked at a health care outpost. There were no hospitals or clinics out here. This outpost was all the people had. Prior to my arrival, one man had been tasked with taking care of the thousands of people in and around the local village. Now I joined him. I soon saw the misery of poverty.

One day, a woman came to us with a red-hot fever. She was sick with tuberculosis. The man I was working with had no treatment for her. He didn't know what to do.

"Can you send her to Algiers?" I asked.

"No. There's no way. She doesn't have the money. And there's no transport."

"What do we do, then?"

The man came up with an idea. He opened the icebox. He had the woman get in front of it so she could cool off. We didn't have a refrigerator or electricity.

"Oh my God, this is great," she exclaimed.

She was happy to have some relief. The man gave her aspirin, another anti-inflammatory drug, and an injection of vitamins and sent her home. I knew that wasn't going to save her. The man knew it too.

"That's all I can do," he said, voice cracking.

Through this experience, my commitment to medicine was reinforced. It wasn't about rote learning and note-taking. It was about alleviating human suffering.

I returned to the university. In time, I came up with a solution for my note-taking problem. Back in 1968, when I was doing my summer job in the lab for public works, there was a small Roneo (a mimeograph) that was used. It was a poor man's Xerox machine. Good for making copies. I went back and asked my old friends at the lab and the director if I could take the Roneo since they were no longer using it. They gave it to me.

I then pulled together a group of four or five classmates who wanted more time to participate in student politics.

"Listen, guys," I said to them. "Instead of all of us going to every course, what about designating a notetaker for each? They will go to the class, take the notes, and then I will copy them using the Roneo."

I was met with enthusiasm. We began our note-taking plan. I selected the classes that I went to, choosing ones that I liked. I painstakingly took the notes for these classes. The other members of the group took the notes for the other classes. Each class was large enough for one's absence to go unnoticed.

I copied everyone's notes on the Roneo, and then we distributed them. Our system was a success. In time, other students joined. Soon enough, we had about 20 in the group.

I now had extra time to, among other things, study medical textbooks from the French embassy and the library, which I found to be more interesting than going to class. I also had more time to engage in student politics and go to parties. It was wonderful. It wouldn't last, however.

One day, a friend in the note-taking group told me, "I can manage the Roneo if you want. Your apartment is small, especially compared to the house I'm in. Let me take it."

I let him do so. It was a mistake I would soon regret. I wasn't aware that he was a member of the Communist Party, not unlike my other friend, Walkhereddine.

Soon enough, I was arrested by the Sécurité Militaire. They took me in for interrogation. My heart was pounding as they sat me down.

"Are you printing anti-government propaganda?"

"No."

Unconvinced, another one of them replied, "You're printing communist pamphlets. We found the Roneo at your friend's place. He told us you're the one who gave it to him and that you took it from the national lab for quality control. Is that true?"

"I didn't take the Roneo," I insisted. "It was given to me. And it wasn't supposed to be used for printing pamphlets. It was for making copies of notes from class."

My words had little effect. The same interrogators continued to press me.

I spent the night in lockup. Thankfully, I wasn't harassed or subjected to anything worse than the interrogation I had already endured. Unbeknownst to me, two of my distant cousins were top-ranking members of the Sécurité Militaire.

The next day, I was released. My interrogators had come to realize I wasn't guilty. They were confiscating the Roneo, however. Nadia was relieved, as she hadn't heard from me in two days (by now, we were together).

Furious, I called the friend who had been managing the Roneo. I learned that his friends from the Communist Party had asked him to print the pamphlets. Walkhereddine had helped him.

In the days following my arrest, my friend and Walkhereddine distanced themselves from me. They felt I had been released too quickly and suspected I was working for the Sécurité Militaire. Meanwhile, with the Roneo gone, I had to attend all my classes again.

Radiology, Love, and Loss   5

As a medical student, I was rotating at the hospital that my radiologist uncle, Djillali, was working at. He was at the leading edge of interventional neuroradiology research, many years ahead of his time. Students came from all over Europe to study with him.

In 1973, Djillali showed me the first computed tomography (CT) scan of a patient, done by Sir Godfrey Hounsfield, revealing brain structures in an unprecedented way.[1] Although the technology was in its infancy, my uncle correctly insisted that it was going to be a complete revolution.

I was excited by what I saw and by the larger world of radiology. It incorporated my favorite subjects, including mathematics, physics, and biology. This was it! I was going to become a radiologist.

For me to do so, I needed to travel overseas to train. Sweden, the United States, and France were options. My mother forbade me from choosing the latter.

"The French abused us for 132 years. If you go there, they'll abuse you for another 20," she stated.

Ultimately, I chose the United States. To train there, I needed to be certified by the Educational Commission for Foreign Medical Graduates (ECFMG), which meant that I had to pass a medical science exam (the equivalency exam) and an English proficiency test.[2] Dean Abdelmoumene encouraged me to get certified. If I did so, he'd reach out to friends in the United States to help me find a residency. Motivated, I began my preparations.

～

When I entered the medical program at the University of Algiers, Nadia became my classmate. I was older now, and so was she.

During our days at the swim club, we had been acquaintances. Now we gradually became much more. We started to truly understand and know each other. She was intelligent, beautiful, and wonderfully unique.

On January 18, 1969, I invited Nadia to a small party at the apartment I lived in. There, I asked her if she wanted to date me, though not in those exact words. Back then, etiquette was different. Thankfully, Nadia said yes.

When Nadia introduced herself to my mother, the latter recognized Nadia's last name. Nadia's uncle had, long ago, worked in the same political party as my father, and the Azza family was known and respected. This helped Nadia earn my mother's and father's approval.

~

Meanwhile, I continued progressing through medical school, with the dream of completing radiology training in the United States in my mind. The foreign medical graduates commissioned in the United States recommended a list of books to study. I couldn't find any in Algiers.

The American Library in Paris sold them, however. My brother Moustafa, now an engineer building one of the first steel plants in Algeria, sometimes traveled to France for work. I asked Moustafa if he could get the books for me.

"Let me see what I can do," Moustafa replied.

When Moustafa traveled, his company gave him money for expenses. The next time he went to France, he stayed at a friend's place rather than a hotel to help save some of his per diem. Moustafa used this money to buy the books.

He came back and gave them to me. I was shocked to learn that each book cost somewhere between $70 and $100. What Moustafa did was generous, and it spoke volumes about the strength of the Zerhouni family bond.

I now studied directly from the American textbooks. As in my years at Lycee Emir Abdelkader and my childhood during the war, I was educating myself. To understand the textbooks, however, I had to learn English.

Initially, it took me 20 minutes to get through a page of text. With more practice, my reading sped up. To help me learn English, I listened to the BBC.

All the hours spent preparing for the equivalency exam led me to miss classes.

While what I was doing appeared risky, I didn't see it that way. My preparation for the equivalency exam required me to study subject matter I would've been learning in class.

When making a decision that entailed a degree of risk, I always asked myself, what is the worst that could happen? In this case, I might mess up a few of the modules here and there and then need to redo them. I might fail to get the equivalency. These worst-case scenarios were not enough to deter me.

For making decisions, using the worst-case scenario as a partial basis for whether you should proceed is prudent. You have to make sure you can handle the worst potential outcomes. If you can, then why not move forward?

~

For the gastrointestinal module, Nadia agreed to take notes for me. Accordingly, I rarely showed up to class. When I did, I sat next to Nadia. Our disciplinarian teacher, Dr. Illoul, the man who headed the gastrointestinal program, noticed my frequent absences and was not pleased.

On the day of the final exam for the module, I finished the test quickly. I handed it to Dr. Illoul. A week later, Nadia informed me I had failed the exam. In disbelief, I demanded that Dr. Illoul review my written test with me. He refused and called me a cheater. He wanted to have me expelled. I insisted I was innocent.

I appealed to Dean Abdelmoumene to let me take an oral reprieve test, administered by a different instructor. I completed it. Afterward, the instructor, who was impressed by my performance, asked how I had known so many answers.

I told her I had been studying from the American textbooks. She asked me questions that were not covered in the course. I successfully answered them.

She gave me a passing grade, warning, "Don't pull this stunt again."

~

In 1973, one of the saddest episodes of my life occurred. Chahid, the second oldest of my brothers, died. He was only 33, leaving behind two children and a wife. During the war, death had come close, yet it had not touched me like this.

While Chahid was visiting the United States, a friend invited him to Saint Kitts, a Caribbean Island. On the way back from the island, their boat broke down. Chahid tried to swim to shore. He was never seen again.

It was excruciating to be unable to find his body. I had dreams of him alive on an island. In these dreams, I found him and brought him back.

Chahid was nearsighted and wore thick glasses. He was serious and driven. He went to the best schools and was always the top of his class. He was the smartest one in the family.

At the time, Chahid was a high-ranking employee of SONATRACH, Algeria's national oil company, and he had a PhD in aeronautics and operations research, which in those days was as cutting edge as artificial intelligence is today. He had trained in the United States and was a Fulbright scholar.

My father was crushed by his death, though my mother took it the hardest. Years ago, she had lost a daughter. Now she faced this.

She had so much hope for Chahid. While she loved us all, she and he were especially close. Growing up, Chahid's poor vision and the fact that he was not as handsome as the other brothers made him an underdog. My mother protected him fiercely.

Before Chahid's death, my mother was the life of the party, able to make everyone laugh. After his passing, she didn't give as much attention or importance to anything. She withdrew from social life. She didn't want to be bothered anymore. She stopped praying. She wouldn't believe in God.

～

One of the reasons people are religious is to understand mortality and the finality of the world.

Although my father was a Muslim, he felt that Judaism and Christianity were honorable religions. He also thought that one could relate to God directly and that there was no cleric that could speak in the name of God. God was in one's heart.

"You have to follow the path your conscience tells you rather than that which other people order you to follow," my father insisted.

Unfortunately, the Muslim orthodoxy of the time was that if you didn't think like the clerics, you were excommunicated. It was like the Christianity of the Middle Ages. There was intolerance, narrow-mindedness, and backward thinking.

Despite the shortcomings of some Muslims, I had always identified with the religion, which had a countless majority of noble believers in its ranks.

Yet I also didn't quite believe in genuflections and outward signs of religiosity. I was pragmatic, and I didn't support the forcing of religion on individuals or the use of religion to deny scientific progress or gain political power. I wasn't anti-religious, however. I respected what others believed, and I tolerated the differences.

I believed there was a God I could relate to directly. Those who thought there was nothing could not explain how the universe came to exist in the first place. How did we go from zero—no space, no time, no matter—into something? That jump was impossible for a mind to fathom. It was an insurmountable mystery. I had a profound sense of awe about the fact that the universe existed at all.

Yet existence came with pain and loss. Humans were fragile. Our time on Earth was finite. In the span of a breath, we could depart.

~

Out of respect for my brother's passing, Nadia and I delayed getting engaged. At this point, we still weren't. We were two broke, busy medical students.

Nadia's father was visiting their hometown, Sidi Bel Abbès, when he heard a rumor that my mother didn't like Nadia and would never allow me to marry her.

Furious, Nadia's father informed Nadia. Equally furious, Nadia took her car and drove straight to see my mother. Thankfully, it turned out to be just a misunderstanding. While Nadia was satisfied, her father remained displeased.

"You've been going with this boy for three years," he told Nadia. "I know you are students, and you can't get married right now, but people are talking, and I don't know what his intentions are."

I went to visit her father to inform him of my intentions. I dressed up, put a tie on, and arrived at his elegant law office. It was located on one of the biggest avenues in Algiers. I sat in front of his desk, face-to-face with him. A powerful, handsome man, he could've passed for a 1950s movie star.

"You're wearing a tie today," he observed.

"Sir, I have honest intentions with your daughter," I stated. "We love each other. I hope that later, when we can, we'll get married."

"That's nice, but I want to hear from your parents, also."

Later, my father called and assured him. Fortunately, that was enough.

~

I was now in the final stage of the medical curriculum, the internship year. I was to take the equivalency exam in Paris in the spring of 1975, during my neurology clerkship.

I traveled to Paris for the test. I was among around 500 students, from all over the world, speaking many different languages. It was like the Tower of Babel.

I finished the test and wouldn't find out for several weeks whether I passed. In the meantime, I wanted to have fun in Paris. I had friends and a cousin living in the city.

We had a great time. Several weeks passed. I was supposed to be back in Algiers doing my neurology clerkship. I thought my absence would go unnoticed. I was wrong.

Learning that I was in Paris, the head of neurology, Professor Geronimi, sent a disciplinary note to Dean Abdelmoumene.

My brother, Diden, called me and asked me to come back immediately.

I returned to Algiers, and on my way to a disciplinary meeting with Dean Abdelmoumene and Professor Geronimi, I checked my mail. There was an envelope from the ECFMG. I learned I'd passed the equivalency exam by a significant margin. My good feelings were short-lived, however, as I soon met with the dean and Professor Geronimi. It was an interrogation.

"I've never seen disrespect to this extent," Dean Abdelmoumene fumed. "Not even showing up, not even asking for an excuse, not even sending a note, not even . . . I mean, what student does that?"

To make matters worse, the dean remembered the incident where the head of the gastrointestinal program accused me of cheating. Stoking the fires, Professor Geronimi insisted they make an example of me.

"How do you explain you not going to this clerkship?" the dean asked me.

"Sir, if you remember, I came to see you about my future, and I told you I was going to get ready for the U.S. equivalency exam. Well, that's what I was doing."

"For four weeks in Paris?"

"No, but I did take my exam."

"Oh yeah? And how did that go?"

"Actually, I got the results today."

I handed the dean the letter from the ECFMG. He opened it. His eyes widened. His disbelief transformed into joy as he turned to Professor Geronimi. "This is the first goddamn student at our school to get the American equivalency."

"Yeah, yeah, but that's not the issue," Professor Geronimi interjected.

"Professor Geronimi, please. We should honor this student, not kick him out."

I breathed easier. I'd dodged another bullet. The crisis resolved, and moving forward, Dean Abdelmoumene was extraordinarily helpful.

He knew the dean at Johns Hopkins. He knew the dean at Harvard. He knew people at the NIH. Abdelmoumene wrote to them on my behalf.

He received an answer from the Johns Hopkins University School of Medicine and convinced Dr. Russell Morgan, the dean and former radiology chair at Johns Hopkins, to take me on. It would be for only three to six months, and I would need a scholarship from the Algerian government.

The minister of education and the minister of health had decided to build a new hospital. They were giving scholarships out to help train Algerians who would hopefully become the future leaders of the facility. I was offered one.

"Take it and go to the United States," Dean Abdelmoumene insisted.

The government scholarship would be $369 a month. It was a lot of money for them, but it wouldn't be enough to support Nadia and me. Regardless, we would be going. My intention then was not to stay in the United States for good. I wanted to come back and help my country.

In the fall of 1975, Nadia and I completed our training at the University of Algiers and received our medical school diplomas. On October 25, I married Nadia, the love of my life. We honeymooned in Paris and Sweden. In the latter, we visited the wife and children of my deceased brother.

Next, we would journey to the United States. Our flight went through Reykjavik. It was the cheapest one we could find. I was 24 and about to begin a new era in my life, far from friends and family though thankful to have my wife by my side.

AMERICAN DREAM II

Johns Hopkins Radiology 6

Nadia and I arrived in Baltimore in December 1975. My government scholarship of $369 a month would be mailed to me as a check at the end of each month. For now, I had to make do with the few hundred dollars I had in my pocket.

Nadia and I took a cab into Baltimore, anxious to see the city. We were expecting skyscrapers and bright lights. Yet it was dark. The harbor was in ruin. The homeless walked the streets. The city was in shocking disrepair.

"This is Baltimore?" I uttered in disbelief.

"Where did you bring me?" Nadia asked, concerned.

Johns Hopkins University was in the middle of downtown. We arrived at a Sheraton hotel near the Johns Hopkins hospital and medical school. The hotel charged something like $35 a night. We wouldn't be able to afford it for long.

The next day, Nadia and I tried to go for a stroll, wanting to explore the neighborhood. A security guard stopped us.

"Where are you going?" he inquired, confused.

We didn't speak English well, though I knew enough to respond, "To walk."

"You don't walk around this neighborhood."

"Why?"

"Son, do you want to get killed?"

In Algiers I could walk the streets at 2 a.m. without issue. Baltimore, in contrast, was like a war zone, especially around Hopkins. There were gunshots at night. There were abandoned houses with bullet holes in them.

The next day, Nadia and I visited the Hopkins radiology department, which was small. Radiology wasn't a prominent specialty at the time.

At the entrance to the department, a woman named Chris Simmons worked as an assistant and would stay in that role for more than 40 years, appreciated by all. A resident of East Baltimore, Chris was kind, gentle, and diminutive

Nadia and I approached her. Chris understood enough of our broken English to know that she should take us down to Dr. Stanley Siegelman's office.

Stan was the vice chair of the department, and when we entered his cramped office, we found him sitting behind his desk. He began talking to us.

"Speak slowly please," I responded, having difficulty understanding him.

"Oh, you don't speak English very well?" Stan asked.

"Yes. A little bit, sir. I learned English last year."

"I see." Stan was concerned. Eventually, he said, "So, Dr. Morgan sent you to us for a few months, but to be honest, I don't think your English is good enough. Before you begin here, maybe we should send you to the language school to learn some more English."

Fear gripped me. I tried to explain that my scholarship was for only a few months. I was here to learn radiology now, not later. I could read and write and understand enough English to do the program. I begged Stan to let me move forward.

"Let me check with our chair, Dr. Martin Donner," Stan said.

Stan left to go speak with Martin. In time, he returned.

"Okay. Come over and meet our chair."

Nadia and I did so. Martin was friendly, and I learned he was from East Germany. I was far more fluent in German than in English. To Martin's surprise, I began speaking to him in it. We conversed, and I persuaded him to let me proceed with my training.

With Martin's approval, I would join the medical students who were doing a radiology elective. Meanwhile, Nadia would eventually get in touch with Dr. Claude Jean Migeon, director of pediatric endocrinology at Hopkins. The two would connect, as Claude was French and quite kind. Nadia would go on to do a fellowship in pediatric endocrinology, developing friendships with fellows from all over the world, which she enjoyed.

$\sim$

Long before our arrival at Hopkins, in the early 1900s, American medical education needed standardization and reform. Educational theorist Abraham Flexner headed a survey of medical education in the United States, the results of which led to the demise of some inadequate schools and the reform of others.[1] In his report, Flexner used Hopkins as a benchmark for quality.[2] The academic model that Flexner supported and of which Hopkins was the standard-bearer has defined American medical education into the present.[3] A key component of this model is the clinical teaching system. Hopkins professor Sir William Osler developed this innovation in the nineteenth century, ensuring that Hopkins was far ahead of its time and that its students learned at the patient's bedside rather than just through memorizing textbooks.[4]

~

The medical curriculum I had at the University of Algiers was in line with what was done in the United States, and therefore I found no big differential to overcome as I began my training with the Hopkins radiology department. There was a difference in culture, however. As a student, I was used to being silent and obedient, which was the European way. In America, a country of freedom, one was judged by their ideas and questions. I was encouraged to speak up and be more expressive.

Another major difference between Algerian and U.S. medical schools was that, in my homeland, because there were so few medical students, we all obtained much more clinical experience. When we went to the hospital in Algiers, there weren't tons of residents ahead of us. We were the first generation.

Both Nadia and I had worked in the emergency room (ER). We had done minor surgery and helped with child deliveries in all kinds of cases. I had read radiology films, and I had been taught how to take them. I was more practically trained than the medical students at Hopkins.

Regardless, the medical students in the elective were terrific. Stan Siegelman had one of them, Ed Shapiro, be my chaperone. Ed and I became friends (and would also become scientific collaborators in later years).

As the elective progressed, I worked hard to improve my English. Thankfully, I made progress. Listening to the radio and watching TV helped.

Nadia and I were now living next door to the hospital, in an apartment in the famous 550 building, where all the "new guys" went because it was affordable. Even still, the rent was around $200 a month. The only money I had coming in was the $369 I received each month from my government scholarship. Although it was difficult to financially survive, I needed to find a way to live in the United States for only three to six months. After this, I planned to return to Algeria and become a radiologist at the University Hospital of Algiers, which had yet to be built.

In the elective, I met an intelligent faculty member named Paul Wheeler. He loved computers. He thought they were going to revolutionize radiology.

Paul and I developed a good relationship. After my training for the day was done, I stuck around and read films with him. Paul had created an automated language processing system for generating radiology reports. I loved it and worked hard to master it.

Another member of the faculty I bonded with was Bob Gayler. He was the wise man of the department. Everyone went to him when they had an issue. Extraordinarily dedicated, Bob stayed late, helping residents with difficult cases. His calm demeanor was reassuring.

A true gentleman, Bob showed me what it was to be a Johns Hopkins physician: dedicated, hardworking, socially minded, and nondiscriminatory. This lesson in conduct and character extended beyond my role as a doctor, however. It was a way to live.

~

I finished the six-week elective and went into the radiology residency program. I wasn't a formal resident, however. I was still just a visitor without a long-term position, paid only by the Algerian government. Meanwhile, Nadia had learned she was pregnant. Our child was due in August. It was wonderful news, yet if our baby was coming, I needed to be making more money.

The chief resident approached me and asked if I could take on some of the unpopular radiology night shifts at the emergency room. The 12-hour night shift was a paid position.

"Wonderful," I replied. "How many nights can I get?"

I ended up working seven days of night shifts every other week while continuing to fulfill my duties during the day.

The ER was trial by fire, and I was met with the reality of downtown Baltimore. There were gunshot wounds. There was misery. There was death. I kept composed, handling the cases that came my way, interpreting the radiographs, and dictating my observations. I was grateful for the opportunity to help the patients who came in, many of them poor. I was also grateful to have such an excellent supporting cast.

The radiology technician was a Filipino American named Bucco (who, to my recollection, had been in the navy as a corpsman to earn his citizenship). He was funny and the salt of the earth.

In addition to Bucco, there was also Larry Hineline, who sorted the films. Larry was a high school student moonlighting to earn some money.

Kind and capable, he was an invaluable member of our team in an ER that brought forth plenty of unforgettable cases.

One time, a patient came in with a stab wound in his chest. We hurried him to the X-ray room. Bucco took the films, which I then examined. The patient had a collapsed lung. He certainly couldn't go home.

The patient was put on a stretcher in the waiting room beside a man who came into the ER with a cut hand. We didn't know this man was the one who had stabbed the patient. The man had accidentally cut his hand on the knife when he did it.

The two didn't realize they were next to each other until the nurse pulled open the curtain separating them. A fight ensued. Thankfully, we were able to stop it before anyone was killed.

Through the trials of the night shift, I became a better doctor. At Hopkins, there was an unwritten rule that one had to be a great doctor first, then you could be a scientist or a teacher. In my mind, the master clinician Phil Tumulty was an example of the Hopkins standard of excellence.

Phil would demonstrate this excellence in an episode that occurred years later. Through a CT scan, I would diagnose a patient in his thirties with what I thought was testicular cancer. Others would agree with my diagnosis.

Phil would be called in as a consultant. Through spending time with the patient and evaluating him, Phil would question our initial diagnosis. He believed the cancer was pancreatic, despite what the CT scan had indicated. A biopsy would ultimately prove Phil was correct. Yet how had he known?

"Ninety percent of the time, the patients will tell me what they have. I just listen to them."

His words underscored the need for physicians to retain and sharpen their ability to listen to patients regardless of the technology at their disposal. Today, doctors have little time left to listen to patients the way Phil did. Precious minutes during medical visits are largely swallowed up by doctors staring into their computer screens, filling out mandated data fields, all to enable efficient billing and provide documentation to prove they really "listened" to their patients.

The patient, Jad Khouri, whom Phil had correctly diagnosed with pancreatic cancer, would pass on. The patient's brother, Nagi Khouri, a Lebanese radiologist and faculty member at Hopkins, was a dear friend, an exceptional mentor during these early Hopkins years, and an outstanding physician who placed patient care above all. In a career defined by empathy, Nagi made immeasurable contributions to the detection and prevention of breast cancer both in the United States and abroad. He helped provide these services to the elderly and the poor in Baltimore, and as a researcher, he helped pioneer advances that have shaped the world of radiology. Nagi was—and will always be—a shining example of why America must keep its doors open to immigrants of talent.

~

In time, an ER case arrived that provided me with a chance to shine. A patient came in with hip pain. It was a hip fracture. However, the standard films we were required to take didn't clearly show the break. In Algiers, I had learned how to angle the camera in a way that allowed one to definitively see this type of fracture. I took films using this angle, which allowed me to confirm the break.

In the morning, Paul Wheeler came in and, as he always did, checked every ER case to make sure there were no screwups. He examined the standard films for the patient with the hip fracture and looked at my report.

"Where the hell do you see this fracture?" he asked me.

I pointed at one of the standard films. "Don't you see that there's a little buckle?"

Paul looked at it, unconvinced. "You call that a fracture?"

"Yeah. And I'll show you why."

I brought out the films I had taken using the angle I learned in Algiers. On them, the fracture was clearly visible.

"Oh my God. You got it right," Paul responded, impressed.

Through moments like these, Paul came to value my abilities and insisted that I stay on with Hopkins after the end of my training. Yet there was no opportunity for me to do so. Meanwhile, the hospital in Algiers was far from being built, which meant that going home wasn't a good option.

I started applying to radiology programs around the United States. I was accepted at Loma Linda University in California. They offered me a paid residency position. It seemed like a good fit. As I prepared to leave Hopkins, part of me wished I didn't have to.

Thankfully, the Hopkins radiology faculty liked me, and there was a resident who wanted to leave the program. The faculty decided that I would take that resident's place. Stan called and made me the offer. The formal residency program had a regular salary. I gladly said yes.

Residency and a   7
Dying Algerian President

I found the residency program to be case oriented, practical, and intense. The hours were long and demanding. We learned at an extraordinary pace. By the end of the year, a student might have reviewed 2,000 or 3,000 cases, observing numerous diseases and diagnoses.

"Listen," Paul Wheeler said, "being a radiologist is like being a pilot. The pilot who flies 100 hours is not as good as the one who has flown 1,000 hours and even less good than the one who's flown 10,000 hours. So what kind of pilot are you going to be, Elias?"

Paul's lesson underscored a basic principle of success. To be great, you must put in the hours. Without mastering your craft, how can you become a master?

Paul was one of the many terrific professors I had at Hopkins. Fred Stitik and Stan Siegelman were others. In particular, Stan was the most remarkable professor in the program. He demanded much of his students and was a brilliant radiologist in his own right.

While the faculty were outstanding, so were my fellow residents, including David Naidich, whose verbal IQ was extraordinary. We became fast friends and started working together on CT.

I also formed strong relationships with the nurses and technicians. When I was in medical school in Algeria, I had learned how to perform their tasks. During my residency at Hopkins, if a technician or nurse did not know how to do something, I could help them.

"If you don't know how to do something, you have no right ordering other people to do it," my radiologist uncle, Djillali, once told me.

~

As August neared its end, Nadia was overdue with our first child. On September 1 at around 2 a.m., she woke me up. Our baby was coming. I took her to the Johns Hopkins Hospital. She was examined. The doctor said the birth wouldn't happen before 11 a.m.

I had a radiology/pathology conference to lead that morning. Trusting the doctor, I went to it. Around 8:30 a.m., I received an urgent call and learned that I had just missed my son's birth. Upset, I rushed back to be with Nadia. I held her hand and saw my son, Will, for the first time.

Nadia was able to take care of Will, as she didn't have to cover nights. Her fellowship in pediatric endocrinology gave her a degree of control over her schedule.

Nadia's ability to do her fellowship and publish research while raising a family was incredible. She did all this while also being a pillar of strength and support in my life. I couldn't have achieved all I have without Nadia by my side.

The partner one chooses in life can make or break their future. This was a lesson I'd be reminded of often as Nadia supported me throughout the years.

In raising Will, Nadia was helped by Elvie Hineline, the mother of Larry Hineline, the young man who had sorted films as part of my team at the ER. Elvie babysat Will often. She grew to truly love him. Elvie would become a lifelong family friend.

~

Although I'd extended my stay in the United States, I still planned to return to Algeria. The University Hospital of Algiers was supposed to be built by 1979, and my U.S. student visa would end with the completion of my Hopkins training. Knowing I would eventually leave, I wanted to absorb all there was to learn while I had the chance. I doubled down, working hard and staying long hours.

Later in the residency program, one or two of us would be made chief residents. This coveted, prestigious post had two clear front-runners, neither of whom was me. In those days, it was unlikely for a foreign medical graduate to achieve such an honor.

The faculty met and discussed who would become chief resident. Much to my surprise, they chose me in addition to Jay Dobrow. Yet again, Hopkins had proved to be above prejudice.

Meanwhile, I volunteered to work with the first CT scanner at Hopkins, made by Electric and Musical Industries (EMI). Although revolutionary, the EMI scanner was a clunker. It took minutes to do one image, laughable by the standards of the future, where a CT scanner would be able to do one image in 50 milliseconds. When the images came out, I took a Polaroid of them because the scanner had practically no memory. Despite the machine's flaws, I was fascinated by the technology. I learned the nuts and bolts of it.

There was a physicist in the radiology department named Frank Leo, who was collaborating with a company known as American Science and Engineering (AS&E). AS&E had developed a body CT scanner, and among its remarkable virtues, it could obtain images in 10 seconds.[1]

Stan offered me the opportunity to work with the AS&E scanner with him and Frank. The prototype was placed at Hopkins. The AS&E scanner had bugs and broke down frequently. Regardless, it was a thrilling leap forward. By working with the scanner, I put myself in a position to learn new principles of imaging. The lesson here is that exploring new innovations and technologies early is essential.

Stan Siegelman fell in love with the new technology and was going to use the AS&E scanner half the time for body imaging, while neuroradiology would use it the other half. I would be one of Stan's principal assistants, along with David Naidich. Few had done research on CT scanning beyond the head, which gave Stan, David, and me the opportunity to lead in that field.

Stan and I worked on a research project involving pulmonary nodules, which was his idea. In those days, chest surgery, a dangerous procedure, was often performed to distinguish benign nodules from malignant ones. It had been shown through a study at the Mayo Clinic that benign pulmonary nodules contained more calcium than cancerous ones.

Calcium had much higher CT numbers, and Stan wanted to quantify calcium content with a CT scanner to reduce the need for chest surgery. Our project succeeded but was met with controversy, as others could not reproduce our results. This pulmonary nodule research project would be something I'd pursue further in the years after I left Hopkins. For now, it remained an unresolved issue.

～

In the fall of 1978, I still eyed an eventual return to Algeria, even though the construction of the University Hospital of Algiers had yet to be started. To work in my homeland, I had to pass an Algerian equivalency exam.

I traveled to Algiers, arriving on the Sunday before the test was given. The exam would be on Thursday. In the days leading up to it, I visited with family.

On Tuesday morning, I received an urgent call from my radiologist uncle.

"Last night, President Boumediene was admitted to the main hospital," he said.

Boumediene had collapsed. It appeared he'd suffered a stroke. The government asked Djillali to consult. A CT scan needed to be done. Yet Algeria didn't have a CT scanner, and no one could deliver one fast enough.

"Do you have any idea how we can do it, Elias?" Djillali asked.

I remembered how physicist Frank Leo and I had once helped a company that had the idea of putting CT scanners on trucks. Since the company wanted to sell the service to the U.S. Army, the truck was designed so it could be moved by aerial military transport.

"There's a company that has just completed their first portable CT scanner truck," I told Djillali. "It's in San Diego. It can be quickly transported by the Lockheed C-5 Galaxy military aircraft for which it was designed."

Djillali called the Algerian minister of health, informing him of the solution I had. The minister gave us his full support.

I called Frank Leo in Chicago. He helped me get on the phone with the company that had the truck. They agreed to let us use it. However, the Algerian government had to arrange the truck's transportation to Algeria.

The government contacted the White House (Jimmy Carter was president). At the time, Algeria was helping the United States by acting as a go-between country with Iran. Accordingly, the White House ordered a Lockheed C-5 Galaxy to transport the CT scanner to Algiers.

I was woken that morning and informed I had to go into the hospital. The scanner had arrived. At the hospital, it took a few hours to set up the scanner. After the trial tests were completed, it was time to scan Boumediene. I had, long ago, met him briefly at a student event. Back then, he had been a handsome, red-haired, mustached man with penetrating green eyes.

Now, as they brought an unconscious Boumediene in, he was swollen, and his skin was hemorrhaging. Although he was 47 years old, he looked much older. I scanned his head and found he had large hematomas compressing his brain stem.

"If they don't operate in the next few hours, he's going to deteriorate," I told my uncle.

"We have to talk to the doctors and family right away," my uncle said, agreeing with me.

"Yeah, we do. But what does he have?"

My uncle disclosed that the president had a rare blood cancer, Waldenström's macroglobulinemia. The famed Dr. Waldenström was coming to Algiers that day to examine the president.

My uncle and I met with the president's doctors and wife, Anissa. The atmosphere was tense and almost dysfunctional. Both Algerian and Russian doctors were present. Anissa aggressively asked the president's chief of staff, Colonel Alahoum, to leave the room. My sense was she didn't trust him.

She asserted that the Algerian doctors didn't know what they were doing and that Boumediene had told her to trust only the Russians and the Russian doctors. This upset the few Algerian doctors in the room.

One of them, Dr. Toumi, a war veteran, pointedly told her, "He is Algeria's president, not Russia's, my little lady."

My uncle described what we had found through CT, echoing my assertion that if we didn't operate soon, the president would deteriorate.

"I don't think we can do surgery. He's bleeding from everywhere," the chief Russian surgeon advised. "Why don't we wait for Dr. Waldenström? He'll tell us what to do."

No one operated, and I was asked to stay so that I could consult with Waldenström when he arrived. I did so, getting to know the famous physician as a result.

Meanwhile, despite my involvement in the battle to save Boumediene's life, I still needed to take the Algerian equivalency exam. The next day, I took the test, which I would pass.

Afterward, I returned to the hospital, seeing numerous key state officials. They were distraught. For more than a decade, Boumediene had been in charge. Now he was on death's door. When he passed away, a struggle for power would surely ensue.

I ventured back outside the hospital to pick up a medical document from a car. The head of security opened the trunk for me. It was full of guns. This man was ready for a fight.

When I went back inside, I saw Abdelaziz Bouteflika and other officials talking to Boumediene's chief of staff, Colonel Alahoum. In 1999, Bouteflika would become president of Algeria.

"How is the president?" Bouteflika asked Alahoum.

"He's improved."

"Really?" I interjected, surprised.

"Last night at 2 a.m., he moved his fingers and toes," Alahoum replied.

This development led some to believe the president was doing better. I knew that wasn't the case. When one's brain died, their reflexes inverted, causing them to move in a stretching motion.

"He's waking up," Alahoum insisted.

"Are you sure?" I asked, unconvinced.

"Yes. And listen to me, even if he can't speak, he can just wink. That's all we need."

"Even if he wakes up and he can only wink, he's still president?"

"Of course."

This was a crazy republic, I thought. And there was nothing more that I could do for Boumediene. I returned to the United States the next day.

Meanwhile, the president was in a coma for a few weeks before passing away. Boumediene would, into the present, remain Algeria's best president. Under his rule, Algeria became stronger. Unfortunately, his successors would not be of the same caliber, and a civil war would ensue in the 1990s.

At Hopkins, chief residents could choose to stay an additional year as faculty members. I chose to do so, as my research was going well and I needed to build my résumé. Meanwhile, back home, the construction of the hospital in Algiers was still nowhere near starting.

"If you can stay in the U.S., stay in the U.S.," my father advised. "If you come back here, you'll bury yourself in mediocrity."

My father was right, and his words touched on a life lesson. Environment could shape or break one's destiny regardless of their talent.

Heeding my father's words, I stayed at Hopkins and became a faculty member at the end of 1978. I continued to work in CT and planned on getting certified by the American Board of Radiology. Yet to do so, I had to have a recognized specialty. CT didn't count. It was so new that one couldn't receive a degree in it.

I chose thoracic (chest) radiology. Faculty member Fred Stitik, his second-in-command Nagi Khouri, and I worked together, using the AS&E scanner to learn everything there was to know about CT of the chest. Until the AS&E machine had come along, CT scanners hadn't been fast enough to take an image of the lungs in the time that someone could hold their breath. Now they could. It fueled our research.

With my career advancing, Nadia, who was again pregnant, gave birth to our daughter Yasmin on June 19, 1979. This time, I was with Nadia when she gave birth. Yasmin was calm, affectionate, and charming and would grow up to be a top surgeon.

As true Baltimoreans, my children would come to love the city, as would Nadia and I. We realized that contrary to our first impressions, Baltimore had its charms, and it was a great place to live and raise a family. The city—and Hopkins—became our home away from home.

In 1980, my father came for a visit. He'd long since retired from teaching and was now working at SONATRACH (Algeria's national oil company). He was the chief of staff for the president of the company, who was his former student. My father's work required him to travel the world, making deals with different countries for the betterment of Algeria. He was visiting the United States for that reason.

On seeing him, I immediately noticed he'd lost weight, and his skin was sickly pale. It was jarring, as my father was usually in good health.

"What's wrong?" I asked.

"I don't know. I'm having problems with my digestion."

I CT scanned him. He had colon cancer, which was blocking his intestine. Whomever had examined him last missed it on the X-rays. I was upset. I pushed my father to have surgery by famed surgeon John Cameron at Hopkins before the cancer worsened, not caring what it would financially cost me.

My father wasn't insured, so the price was steep. Thankfully, his company's insurance covered the expenses. The company's president wanted to help my father.

The operation was a success. My father quickly recovered, regaining his appetite and color. For now, his health was good.

~

By 1980, it was clear that Nadia and I would not be moving back to Algeria anytime soon. Construction on the hospital in Algiers still hadn't started. Additionally, I had gone to Algeria and looked for a position and come away without one despite having helped with the medical care of Boumediene and having offered to bring CT technology into the country.

Thankfully, my career in the United States continued to grow. I was building a future, and I'd started to receive recognition for my work in CT.

In life, if one wanted to surf, it wasn't just their skill that mattered but also the wave they rode. Timing is everything. I was riding a huge wave of computerized medicine. I was participating in the golden era of radiology.

In 1980, Stan Siegelman was invited to speak at an international conference in Rome on body CT, called CARVAT. Stan knew the notable radiologist who ran the conference. Stan had told him about the great work we were doing in CT of the body, imaging the pancreas, liver, blood vessels, and so on. We were some of the first in the world to do what we did.

Both Stan and his wife were not feeling well, and he proposed that I go and speak in his place. I would be a keynote speaker. I couldn't turn it down. Nadia took the children to Algiers first so that they could stay with her parents. Then she joined me in Rome for the conference. My uncle, Djillali, attended as well.

It was my first international conference. I gave several talks. My international reputation was propelled upward. I would be invited to more events. My uncle was proud of me.

The last day of the conference, a friend of his invited us all to a dinner. It was a lovely time. My uncle looked a little tired, though nothing seemed off. He appeared happy and healthy. The next day, he, his wife, and Nadia flew to Algiers.

Meanwhile, I went back to the United States, as I had to take the final board exam. A few days later, I received a call from Nadia. There was a rumor going around that my uncle was quite sick. I was confused; he had seemed fine when I last saw him.

I later found out my uncle had gone jogging and started having chest and belly pain. The next day, he had a massive heart attack. At the hospital in Algiers, they didn't know how to manage heart attacks of this kind. I tried to help them over the phone.

My uncle was transferred to a hospital in France. Two days later, he passed away. It had been only a week since I last saw him. And he was only 51 years old, not unlike his father, who had died at the age of 49 from what we thought was a heart attack. Closer to the present, Djillali's son would also die suddenly, at the relatively young age of 60.

Djillali was an invaluable mentor and a brilliant radiologist. Everyone from Europe came to his department to train because he had mastered vital interventional radiology techniques. He was a respected leader of the Algerian medical community. He was a freedom fighter who had sacrificed for his country.

His death was the second most painful one I had experienced, after that of my brother, Chahid. Yet I was also happy to have made my uncle so proud of me, to have given him such joy, during his final days.

My uncle was buried, and I said good-bye. His death broke one of the strong remaining links I had with Algeria, decreasing the likelihood I would return. Meanwhile, I had created new links in America, and Hopkins remained my home away from home.

There were few institutions in the world that stood above all others. Johns Hopkins was one of them. It had given me opportunities, mentorship, and a promising future. I would forever feel monumental gratitude toward this institution and its people.

In early 1981, however, I would leave Hopkins. Fred Stitik had become chair of the radiology department at Eastern Virginia Medical School in Norfolk, and he would recruit me to be his vice chair. This would be a crucial era in my life, one of new friendships, challenges, and breakthroughs, an era that would transform my future.

Eastern Virginia Medical School and Becoming an Entrepreneur and Inventor

8

There were multiple reasons why I left Hopkins to become vice chair of the radiology department at Eastern Virginia Medical School (EVMS) and DePaul Hospital. I was close to Fred Stitik and enjoyed working with him. He was offering support for my research and a tripling of my income. Meanwhile, my visa was going to expire.

Fred discussed my visa issue with his accountant, Bruce Holbrook, an intelligent man in his early thirties with an unflinching dedication to his clients. Bruce would become a lifelong close friend and adviser.

"The only way Elias is getting a permanent residency visa is if he is shown to be an individual of extraordinary ability and not replaceable by anybody else," Bruce told Fred.

In those days, expertise in CT was rare, and my services were needed. Accordingly, I would ultimately obtain my visa. Bruce worked with the Virginia Employment Commission, which asked him to write the job description for the position of vice chair. In doing so, Bruce underscored the unique skill set that was needed for the role.

Years later, on reflecting on the visa process I'd gone through, Bruce would rightly assert that the United States needed to help make visas more accessible for foreign PhD and medical school graduates educated in the country. These graduates could contribute to the United States in meaningful ways and have a huge impact on American medicine and science.

As Bruce would say, "If America is helping provide and pay for the science and medical education of immigrants of talent, our country needs to let them stay and contribute rather than allowing their talents to go elsewhere."

Prior to accepting the job at EVMS, I'd told Fred that Nadia needed to be able to complete her residency. Fred reached out to the chair of the pediatric department at Children's Hospital of The King's Daughters and secured an interview for Nadia. The interview went well, and she was offered a residency.

~

I officially became vice chair of radiology at EVMS and oversaw the spearheading of emerging technologies throughout the department. The pay for my new job was great. My family and I bought a new house. During the day, while Nadia and I were at work, a woman we hired looked after Will and Yasmin and helped maintain our home.

Her name was Huyn. She was from South Vietnam. Her husband, an officer in the South Vietnamese military, had been killed by the Viet Cong. Huyn had escaped Vietnam with her children. Having myself lived in a war-torn country, I felt for her.

Huyn had a will of steel. She was also kind and gentle, and my children loved her. She was a wonderful mother to her own children as well, emphasizing education.

Huyn's life is a lesson in the value of resilience. No matter the circumstances, she never gave up. We can learn a great deal about resilience and problem-solving by watching how immigrants come to the United States and establish or reestablish their families.

~

In my new job, I returned home at more normal hours and spent more time with my children. In the evenings, after Huyn went home and while Nadia was on night calls for her residency, I looked after Yasmin and Will. I read them stories and put them to bed, treasuring every moment.

I didn't want my children eating fast food or carryout, so I cooked for them. I made pasta. I also made eggs, and I boiled corn. I wasn't a great cook, and the children hated my cuisine.

Our new house had a small pool in which I taught Yasmin and Will to swim. It was wonderful to share an activity with them that I loved. Sometimes, as we played in the pool, I would pretend to be one of Will's favorite movie characters, such as Superman or Jabba the Hut from *Star Wars*.

I taught my kids to swim to protect them from drowning. When Nadia and I had bought our new house, we hadn't been aware that the previous owner's two-year-old daughter had drowned in the lake next to it. When we found out, we were horrified.

Yasmin was two. Will wasn't much older. To keep them away from the lake, I told them frightening stories. I said there were monsters in it who snatched babies.

~

As vice chair, I had a laboratory. I was allowed to use about 20 percent of my time for my own research. I wanted to obtain grants from the NIH, yet the agency and its many institutes (with specific scopes of focus, such as the National Cancer Institute or the National Heart, Lung, and Blood Institute) were not receptive to technological developments. I needed to prove they were directly applicable to a disease that was within the mandate of a given institute.

I continued my research on pulmonary nodules, using a General Electric (GE) CT scanner. I realized that the software that companies were using for CT scanners wasn't standardized. Different scanners gave different numbers. It was a mess.

To help solve this problem, I came up with the idea of a pulmonary nodule reference phantom[1] (a finely engineered object that would be scanned). If one CT scanned a patient's pulmonary nodule and then the pulmonary nodule reference phantom, a density comparison could be done, leading a doctor to determine whether the nodule was likely benign or malignant.

I made the first successful prototype of the pulmonary nodule reference phantom in our garage, using Nadia's pots and pans and pressure cooker. I felt my invention needed to be manufactured immediately.

I went to major companies, including GE and Siemens, and was turned down because surgeons were their biggest customers, and my device would prevent surgeries. The rejections discouraged me. I wasn't sure how to move forward. Meanwhile, I felt deep sadness at the thought of the thousands of patients undergoing needless lung surgery.

Bruce Holbrook visited DePaul Hospital and after reviewing the phantom's applications insisted we get the invention into the marketplace as soon as possible. I informed him about my lack of success with the major companies.

"What do I do now?" I asked Bruce.

"Elias, you're in America. You start your own company."

I had some of the funds needed to pull it off, as the radiology practice was booming. Accordingly, I wanted to put my money toward helping patients. The only problem was that I didn't know how to create a company.

"I'll help you create it," Bruce offered.

Computerized Imaging Reference Systems (CIRS) was born. Our vision was to calibrate and harmonize all computerized imaging with the phantom technology. My first entrepreneurial adventure had begun.

I was too busy to run CIRS on my own. The company needed help—and an office. We recruited Bill Drury, a recently retired navy officer, to act as a manager and help with the mechanics of running CIRS. We also recruited my older brother, Moustafa, as chief engineer.

In these early stages of CIRS, we were developing the materials needed for manufacturing the phantom. Moustafa and Bill had to figure out how to produce an effective phantom with a plastic system that could be replicated and sold. It was trial and error. It involved putting together many little parts, molding them, and then testing what had been made.

Despite the challenges, they ultimately succeeded. A reproducible phantom was made. Unfortunately, the prediction of the companies who had rejected my pulmonary nodule reference phantom idea turned out to be correct. We couldn't sell many. Radiologists didn't buy it because they didn't want to anger referring surgeons.

Meanwhile, a multicenter study that could prove the effectiveness of the phantom (a device now known as the Lung Nodule Reference Simulator) was ongoing. The study included 10 institutions, with Duke University; the University of California, San Francisco; and the Mayo Clinic among them.[2] The study's results could help CIRS if the company could survive long enough. We were almost bankrupt.

The first lesson of a start-up is to have more money than anticipated as well as good advisers. Thankfully, I had the latter.

"Nobody wants to buy the phantom," I lamented to Bruce. "We don't have a product we can sell, and we are running out of money."

"Is there any other application we can pursue?" Bruce asked.

Pharmaceutical companies were developing drugs to treat osteoporosis but were unable to accurately measure the amount of calcium in bone and therefore could not confirm that their medicines worked. Understandably, the Food and Drug Administration (FDA) was reluctant to approve these drugs without such data.

Was it possible to adapt our technology to measure calcium in bone? Soon enough, we created a phantom for osteoporosis that measured calcium in the spine and hips. Its success saved CIRS. With this second product, we learned to be a radiological engineering company, expanding into quality control systems for all radiological applications. We received requests from all over the world, for all kinds of different phantoms.

The multicenter study involving the pulmonary nodule reference phantom was completed in 1985 (and published in 1986),[3] showing that the device worked. Insurance companies mandated the reference phantom test be done prior to their authorizing surgery. This was at a time when insurance companies were trying to protect themselves from excessive medical expenses through the practice of pre-authorization. This was a fundamental paradigm shift in American medicine that led to a future where insurance companies would largely determine what treatment patients would receive. At the time, few realized that the decision-making power would increasingly pass from the providers of care to the payers of care, who would indirectly control the practice of medicine, often to the detriment of patients.

Meanwhile, the demand for the pulmonary nodule reference phantom grew. Lives were saved. The future of CIRS was bright. Our products helped with medical training and pioneered quality control in radiology. We had a "customer matters culture." Listening to them—and meeting their needs—was paramount.

~

As the company slowly scaled up, the strength of new talent would empower its journey forward. Mark Devlin, who would join CIRS in 1991 as Bill's understudy, would be indispensable. Hardworking, sharp, and dynamic, Mark would take over as president after Bill retired, ensuring that CIRS continued its climb toward greater success despite the limited involvement on my part. CIRS would come to have a team of more than 80 employees and generate more than 250 invaluable products, with substantial annual revenue. The company would eventually be acquired by Mirion Technologies, in a move that would bolster its future.

In looking back on the success of CIRS in its earliest years, the company couldn't have succeeded without Moustafa's masterful engineering or without Bill Drury's decisive, dedicated, and frugal management. Bruce Holbrook's help was also instrumental as a gutsy adviser, visionary, and friend. He showed me the American way of entrepreneurship, of which I'd known little.

There were many lessons that I took away from my experience with CIRS. One was to not give up, even if the present circumstances seemed hopeless. There were times when it seemed like we wouldn't succeed, yet we trusted in our vision and kept moving forward. Another lesson was the importance of understanding what the customer wanted and truly listening to them. This ought to be the foundation of any company.

I also learned that there were times when one could be too early with a product, no matter how revolutionary it was. A scientific solution to an unmet need would not always be embraced by the market, especially if financial incentives were not aligned. Finally, I observed the value of leading with a sense of urgency.

A CT Microscope $\qquad$ 9

Under the presidency of Chadli Bendjedid, Algeria was declining. There was rampant corruption. With the religious extremists growing in power, my father predicted civil war.

My father visited me in the early 1980s. He was ill, and I did a CT scan of him. I realized the cancer that had been removed from his colon had spread to his liver. I was devastated.

Time passed, and while my father was visiting Paris for work, I received an urgent call from my brother, Diden.

"Dad isn't doing well," Diden said. "He's dizzy. Something's wrong."

"Make sure they do a CT scan of his head."

They did. The cancer had spread to his brain.

I traveled to Paris and helped with my father's care in the hospital. His health was deteriorating. It was unbelievably painful to witness. My father would eventually leave the hospital, however. To return to Algiers. To go home.

The last time I saw him was at the airport. He was in a wheelchair.

"I don't know if I'll see you again, son, but I don't want you to move back to Algeria. Your brother is with you now. Don't come back. People will soon be killing each other there."

My father died a few months later, in April 1983. He was 69 years old. I would forever miss him. His wisdom and love had shaped my life. He'd raised me in a home of math and science, a gift for which I'd always be grateful.

~

At DePaul, the GE CT scanner I was using couldn't do what the AS&E scanner at Hopkins did because of its software. The software that companies were using for CT scanners wasn't standardized. Different scanners gave different numbers. My research on pulmonary nodules had illuminated this.

I called Morry Blumenfeld, a talented GE executive who helped guide the research and development of the company's CT scan business, which he had aided the launch of.[1] At this point, I had already made my first pulmonary nodule reference phantom in my garage, yet I hadn't founded CIRS.

"There's something wrong with your scanner," I told Morry.

"There is?"

"You can't do what we've been able to do with the Hopkins AS&E scanner and I know why. It's because you're using the wrong approach to get the numbers. You're getting the image right, but the numbers are inaccurate."

Morry suggested I come up to GE for a visit. I did so and presented the work I'd done. The executives were impressed, Morry among them.

"What do you need?" he asked.

"If I had a computer with access to the code and the scanner, I could solve the problem with the latter," I asserted.

Morry offered me an image analysis computer that GE sold with its scanners. If I accepted it, they'd also give me a grant to do research with them and show them how to fix their scanner. I happily said yes. GE shipped the machine to Virginia that afternoon.

I would now have a powerful scanner analysis computer at my disposal, after a single visit of a few hours with Morry.

The outcome spoke volumes about Morry. I was a young scientist with an idea, and rather than shutting me down, Morry had said "why not?"

This experience helped me develop a philosophy of "why not?" that I'd carry with me throughout my life. One should never say "why?" to a child, a young scientist, an artist, or someone else with a big idea. They ought to say "why not?" instead. I realized I had to find colleagues and mentors who shared my philosophy.

I also had to find and work with those who could truly say yes to things, meaning they could actually make them happen. In an organization, there was often a thousand points of veto, numerous people who could not say yes and very few who could and would. Identifying the Morry Blumenfelds of the world and reaching out to them is a key to success.

~

The GE scanner analysis computer arrived, and I began my research on it. They wanted to know what they needed to do to improve it. I found answers that led to new applications.

The slices the scanner was taking were too thick. CT scanners provided a complete picture through slices of images, not unlike using a knife to look into an apple slice by slice. If one had a pulmonary nodule that was 5 millimeters and they took a 1-centimeter slice, they were not cutting into the nodule. I adjusted the GE scanner and the software to take thinner slices and higher-resolution images and obtain accurate numbers. Morry was happy.

When taking a very thin slice of the lung and improving the resolution, one could see details that couldn't be seen before. It was like looking through a microscope. This was high-resolution CT.

It could be used to diagnose lung conditions that had evaded imaging. For example, in Norfolk, many who had worked in the naval shipyards suffered from asbestosis. They were always fighting in court to try to prove they had it. Using high-resolution CT, asbestosis could be elucidated.

~

Although I'd left Hopkins, I worked with Stan Siegelman and David Naidich on a book titled *Computed Tomography of the Thorax*. In it, I shared my research on the pulmonary nodule and high-resolution CT.

In terms of other Hopkins scientists I worked with, there was also the gifted pathologist Ralph Hruban. Robert Heitzman, one of the leading chest radiologists in the world, who'd authored the notable books *The Lung: Radiologic-Pathologic Correlations* and *The Mediastinum: Radiologic Correlation with Anatomy and Pathology*,[2] had found a way to inflate lungs (obtained from autopsies) and then preserve them in that state. I asked Ralph Hruban if we could do this at Hopkins. He said yes.

We studied our newly preserved, inflated lungs. We proved that one could significantly better diagnose diseases of the lung with a CT scanner rather than a regular X-ray machine. Through this research, I used high-resolution CT to differentiate diffuse lung diseases.

~

Fred Stitik invited Robert Heitzman to give a keynote lecture at EVMS. After his lecture, he looked at my work. Using the GE scanner analysis computer, I showed him high-resolution CT images of the lungs. Heitzman insisted that I had to present my work.

"Nobody has invited me to," I replied.

"Because they don't know what you're up to. I mean, I had no idea you were doing this."

A few weeks later, there would be a meeting of the chest radiology societies. All the rock stars of the specialty would be speaking at it, including Tony Proto, Heitzman, and George Genereux. I hadn't been invited.

A week before the meeting, due to a hospitalization, a replacement speaker was needed. Heitzman suggested my name.

"Would you be able to come to Boston next week to present your work?" he asked me.

I excitedly agreed. I flew to Boston.

Soon, I stood on a podium in front of the entire world of chest radiology. In my presentation, I offered a new approach to lung disease. Using a CT scanner as a high-resolution microscope, one could unravel the pathology they saw. I showed high-resolution images of cancer spreading in the lungs. I showed asbestosis and lung fibrosis cases.

Many were amazed. Yet not everyone was supportive. Ben Felson, considered the father of chest radiology, spoke after I was finished.

"It's beautiful work, but it's useless. Why use a several-hundred-dollar, expensive test like CT to look at a lung disease when you can do so with a $30 X-ray and come up with the same diagnosis? That is, if you know how to interpret it, Dr. Zerhouni," Felson jabbed.

Insulted, I shot back, "When I make these high-resolution images, my residents can easily read them. I appreciate that you, Dr. Felson, don't need them, but it takes a long time for one to reach your level of training. Unless we can clone you, it won't be possible for our entire community to read these things properly."

Felson was caught off guard, as were others. I had challenged him. Friends told me I'd likely ruined my career by doing so.

Despite Felson's opposition, there were a lot of young radiologists who were interested in high-resolution CT and wanted me to show them how to do it. Although CT was pricey, the scans were going to get cheaper as we further developed the technology.

In time, there was an explosion of papers on high-resolution CT. I became a recognized innovator for the pulmonary nodule and for looking at lung pathology.

Renowned Duke radiologist Carl Ravin called me to inform me that I had been elected to the Fleischner Society. This prestigious society for thoracic radiology (international in its reach and exclusive, limited membership) allowed me to connect with the world of top-notch chest radiologists and other experts in lung diseases. It was a transformative experience.

When it came to being elected, my supporters had included Fleischner Society members such as Robert Heitzman and, of all people, Ben Felson.

"Zerhouni's got guts," Felson had asserted. "I like him."

~

At EVMS, we would introduce dynamic ultrasound technology. I looked at companies making leading-edge ultrasound equipment. I visited one in Seattle, Advanced Technology Laboratories, which had made a brilliant ultrasound device. With it, one could see things in real time. It was an impressive machine.

I always personally tested any machine we were looking at, so, while in Seattle, I tested this one. Through the process of doing so, the technician spotted a tumor in my thyroid. This was bad news, yet I didn't let it spoil my impression of the machine. We ended up buying it.

When I returned to Norfolk, a surgeon examined my thyroid tumor. Biopsy couldn't prove if it was benign or malignant. Yet at my age, tumors like these tended to be malignant. The surgeon advised that I have it removed.

Through surgery, half my thyroid was cut out, along with the tumor, which turned out to be benign.

"I got operated on for nothing," I vented.

"No, it's not for nothing," the pathologist responded. "These things can be benign now, but 10 years down the line, it could have turned malignant."

Although the surgery averted a potential danger, I felt that it also caused harm. The anesthesia did something to my brain. My memory was partially damaged. For example, I could not remember phone numbers, whereas before, I did not even have to write them down.

~

When my father died, my family and I visited Algeria and grieved with my relatives. At one point, while sitting with my mother, she told me about a health issue she'd been having.

"It's like I have something crushing my chest. I don't know if I ate something wrong or?"

"How often does it come?"

"When I go up the stairs, I feel it."

"It's your heart."

I was concerned. Her older brother Djillali had died of a heart attack, and her father had died from what seemed to be the same thing.

My mother came to Virginia with me so I could evaluate her. Testing revealed a significant narrowing of my mother's left coronary artery. Yet I didn't want her to have open-heart surgery. It came with too many risks.

I wanted her to utilize interventional radiology and do an angioplasty (a minimally invasive way of unblocking a narrowed artery) using a balloon catheter technique developed by Dr. Andreas Gruentzig in Switzerland.[3] Gruentzig, who was now at Emory University, agreed to see my mother the next week. Tragically, a few days before the appointment, Gruentzig died in a plane crash. Yet there was a young cardiologist at Hopkins, Jeff Brinker, who had trained with Gruentzig. He agreed to treat my mother. The procedure was a success.

If this technology had not been invented, my mother would have had to undergo riskier open-heart surgery. It dawned on me that surgery would increasingly become less invasive, yet forwarding this evolution would require innovators to work with engineers and material scientists not typically present in academic centers. Barriers between these disciplines would need to be removed.

~

Meanwhile, Stan Siegelman wanted me back at Hopkins. He offered me a position as codirector of body CT and director of the new magnetic resonance imaging (MRI) division. MRI was a huge part of the future. At EVMS, I wouldn't have access to it.

"I know nothing about MRI," I told Stan.

"I'm aware. There are few radiologists out there who are qualified. This is a new field, but knowing you, I'm sure you'll learn fast enough and come up with something."

If I returned to Hopkins, my salary would be roughly one-third of what it was at EVMS, though the work would be more rewarding. To complicate matters, Nadia had finished her residency and now worked as a pediatrician. She loved her job and had received offers for others in the area. A third child was on the way too.

I called Bruce and asked him for advice.

"Even though EVMS has been good to you and it's an excellent institution, Elias, your career here is not going to support your full intellectual and scientific potential. EVMS doesn't yet have the financial backers of a research institution like Hopkins nor the researchers to collaborate with. Go back to Hopkins. I think you could be an NIH director one day."

~

I couldn't truly make a decision without discussing it with Nadia first. She worried about abandoning her job and my taking such a big pay cut since we had two children to provide for and another one on the way. Protecting them was what mattered most to her. She didn't want to sacrifice their well-being and education. After more discussion, she eventually agreed to let me take the offer.

"As long as you find the children great private schools to continue their education, I'll go along with it."

So that's what we did. By the late spring of 1985, I had officially accepted Stan's offer. I would start at Hopkins on July 1. The pay cut was daunting, yet, thankfully, CIRS was stable and making some money.

On May 11, my son Adam was born in Virginia at the hospital where Nadia worked, bringing joy into our lives. Nadia and I decided to put off the move to Baltimore until after the summer, when our new house would be ready. We didn't want to move baby Adam so soon. We wanted to let him grow. For the time being, I made things work by traveling between Virginia and Baltimore.

I'd taken a large pay cut, yet it was a risk I never regretted, as it would open the door to countless opportunities. In our society, where money earned is often a chief consideration for any job we choose, it can be counterintuitive to realize that some high-paying roles can rob us in the long run.

Returning to Hopkins: President Reagan, Research, and Academic Battles

10

In July 1985, not long after returning to Hopkins, I received a call from Patty Brantley, a navy physician and brilliant former resident of mine at EVMS and DePaul Hospital. Dynamic, intelligent, and kind, Patty was a radiologist at Bethesda Naval Medical Center and was aware of my work with pulmonary nodules and high-resolution CT.

"How available are you to consult for a VIP we have?" Patty inquired, concerned. "The patient has pulmonary nodules, and we're not sure if they are benign or malignant."

"I'd be happy to help. Just tell me when and how."

Later, Patty called me again.

"I just talked to my chief," Patty informed me. "He's agreed to have you come in as a consultant to the medical team of the president."

President Ronald Reagan had been hospitalized. After they had operated on him for his colon cancer, they had discovered pulmonary nodules. They were afraid that it was metastatic disease, meaning that the cancer had spread to his lungs.

In those days, if one had metastatic cancer, life expectancy could be a few months. Some of the president's doctors wanted to operate on the nodules immediately. Yet open-heart surgery was dangerous, and the president was in his mid-seventies, which only added to the risk. Perhaps noninvasively determining whether the president's nodules were benign could help him avoid the procedure.

"We're reaching out to you because you wrote the paper on how to do it on any scanner," Patty said.

As a consultant to the president's medical team, the work was under complete confidentiality. A member of the Secret Service arrived at the radiology department's CT section at Hopkins.

"Where's Dr. Zerhouni?"

"I'm him," I responded.

"Could you give me your driver license and a credit card? We need to vet you."

He left and came back an hour later. I'd passed the vetting.

"Okay, sir. Can you come with me? We're going to Bethesda Naval Medical Center."

I informed Nadia that I had to go to Washington. I couldn't tell her why. I then hopped into the Secret Service car and was driven to the hospital.

At Bethesda Naval Medical Center, I met with the president's physician. Then the chief of the president's medical team came to see me. There was division within the team, with some asserting that they needed to operate on the president's chest immediately and others believing that they needed to wait.

"Can I look at all the president's X-rays?" I asked.

I did so and observed that the president had a few small pulmonary nodules. We needed to do a CT scan.

"Listen," I said to the chief of the medical team. "I need to examine the president directly because I need to figure out exactly where the pulmonary nodules are and how to do the CT scan properly."

"That's fine, Dr. Zerhouni."

I entered the radiology department and waited for the president. A member of the Secret Service arrived, followed by President Reagan. Tall and blue-eyed, the president was a handsome man.

Reagan looked at the nurse and then the technician. "Oh, you two again. We're going steady now. We're going steady," he said with a chuckle.

I was told the president wore hearing aids and I needed to stand in front of him when talking to him. I introduced myself, following these directions, and we began the examination.

We brought him next door to the CT scanner. He sat down on the scanner with ease despite having recently been operated on. The machine took 10 seconds to obtain an image, so the president was going to have to hold his breath for that long. It was a requirement that might not be easy for a 74-year-old.

"Mr. President, for this test, I'm going to teach you how to breathe."

"Son, at my age I know how to breathe," Reagan responded playfully.

RETURNING TO HOPKINS   69

The president was able to easily hold his breath during the scanning. He was still in very good physical shape. When I informed him we were finished, he did not need any help coming out of the scanner and stood up with the strength of a younger man. He asked me if he could see his images on the scanner. They were not ready yet, so I told him that it would not be possible.

"Sounds just like what they told me in my movies. They could never show me the takes right away," he replied.

Later, I analyzed the pulmonary nodules and determined that, thankfully, they were not malignant. They were probably scarring from the time the president was shot. I entered a room where the president's medical team and First Lady Nancy Reagan waited. The atmosphere was tense. I informed them of the news.

"Well, the young doctor says it's not cancer, so we can wait," Nancy Reagan asserted.

"Yes," I said. "You can wait because, if I'm right, in six weeks when you do a follow-up, the nodules will not have changed. If it's cancer, they will have grown. And I don't think six weeks will make a difference."

The medical team agreed to a follow-up in six weeks. President Reagan was released from the hospital with a relatively clean bill of health. For the next few months, he came back every six weeks to have the nodules checked on. I was shown his updated imaging and observed no change. Eventually, we no longer needed to do the checkups.

I received a letter from the president's secretary thanking me for my services. The president and his wife were grateful.

Despite the confidentiality of what I'd done for President Reagan, which I would adhere to, word of my service reached Hopkins. Dick Ross, the dean of the medical school, found out. He called me up.

"We're proud of you. But you should have told me."

"Well, sir, they told me not to speak to anyone."

"I'm not anyone. I'm your dean."

~

Returning to Hopkins in the summer and eventually moving back to Baltimore in the fall was a transition for my family. For Nadia, it was the hardest. To practice in Maryland, she had to get her state medical license. The demands of the process were extensive. It would take two years for her to resume her medical career. Her sadness during this time was countered by the joy of raising our new baby, Adam.

Meanwhile, my return to Hopkins wasn't as smooth as I thought it would be. The nature of my new position was an issue. I was codirector of body CT and codirector of MRI. While a chair might think it was a great idea to have codirectors for a division, appointing two great people to, in theory, serve as two great engines, the reality was the opposite. Having codirectors created conflict about who decided what for the division and about who had the final word.

Whether it is codirectors or co-CEOs, sharing responsibilities like this is a bad idea. The buck has to stop somewhere. Just as the old adage says that a person cannot serve two masters, in addition, two masters cannot lead one organization.

When it came to my co-directorships, body CT wasn't the issue. For CT, I was codirector alongside the brilliant Elliot Fishman. In a long, transformative career, Elliot's contributions to medical imaging, including CT and 3D imaging, would be enormous. From trailblazing with Pixar in the early days of 3D imaging to trailblazing interactive 3D rendering, Elliot would achieve an excellence worthy of Hopkins.

The conflict for me was in the MRI division. I'd been under the impression I was going to be in charge, yet Hopkins had recruited another radiologist to lead alongside me. She was a professor, while I was an associate professor. She assumed she was in charge. I insisted we were coequal. Regardless, I continued my clinical work and research in MRI.

~

Using a radio frequency pulse, an MRI changed the magnetization of what was being scanned. It was almost like radar. One sent a signal and then received the signal back. When one received the signal back, it took time to demagnetize, or relax. The relaxation time could vary, depending on what had been magnetized.

For example, water's relaxation time was a matter of seconds. In contrast, a solid tissue like bone had a relaxation time that was just milliseconds. The shorter the relaxation time, the weaker the signal. The weaker the signal, the lower the signal on the MRI.

We already knew that cancer had a different relaxation time than the tissues it was a part of. Therefore, we decided to use MRI to assess a tumor's response to treatment. In those days, if one treated a tumor, to know if the therapy had worked, one relied on the natural reveal of time. This was suboptimal. I started working with Ralph Hruban, the Hopkins pathologist who had helped me with pulmonary imaging research.

"Ralph, I'd like to image cancer removed from patients. What do we have that we could look at?"

There were fresh prostates available for research because Dr. Patrick Walsh, the famous and brilliant Hopkins urologist, had developed a nerve-sparing surgical technique to remove the prostate, and he received numerous patients from all over the world. Before these prostates were taken to be frozen and sectioned, we imaged them with MRI and discovered something interesting.

Conventional wisdom dictated that prostate cancer imaged through MRI should exhibit a high signal, and the normal prostate tissue should have a lower signal. We observed the opposite. Ralph and I would receive an NIH grant for high-resolution imaging of prostate cancer. My first series of NIH grants were significant. They gave me the ability to build my laboratory.

We looked at lymphomas and rectal cancer. We could track their evolution. The tumors that were sterilized became fibrous and dark, whereas residual cancer was of a higher signal.

I also did MRI on blood vessels. One of the problems was that the scanners were too slow. They couldn't do real-time imaging. I worked on the issue, helping bring about improvements. This gave us additional grants from the NIH.

~

One day, I received a visit from Jim Weiss, the director of echocardiography at Johns Hopkins Hospital. He was a worldwide expert on cardiac mechanics with ultrasound. We knew each other from my radiology training.

"Mike Weisfeldt sends me," Jim said.

Mike Weisfeldt was the head of cardiology. He was considered one of the top cardiologists in the world, a leading-edge thinker who explored novel areas. He had assembled the interventional cardiology division, and he believed MRI was going to be a huge change in cardiology.

"We need your help, Elias," Jim stated.

"How?"

"We need to correlate what we see in MRI with what we know from ultrasound and X-rays. We can't do it because we don't have a marker that's visible by all three. Could you come up with an idea for that?"

"You mean like something you'd attach to the heart?"

Jim responded with a yes. They wanted me to join their team and do research in cardiovascular MRI. At the time, in most institutions, radiologists and cardiologists were like oil and water. They were intensely competitive and often didn't work well together.

Soon enough, Mike Weisfeldt reached out to me directly. He mentioned a radiologist named Bill Brody, who was working at Stanford. I'd heard about Bill before, though I didn't know him personally. To my knowledge, Bill was a talented cardiovascular radiologist who had been at the NIH.

"Bill Brody cofounded a small company called Resonex," Mike told me. "They've created a wide-open MRI machine."

Back then, most MRI machines were narrow, and most couldn't scan the body. Mike loved the idea of a wide-open machine. One could see the heart and intervene on it at the same time. With the Resonex machine, MRI offered a safer alternative to the interventional cardiology done under damaging X-rays.

Mike wanted to bring the machine to Hopkins, to become a center of interventional cardiovascular MRI. To avoid internal conflict, he was willing to have the machine placed at Hopkins's secondary hospital, the Francis Scott Key Medical Center, run by a gifted administrator, Ron Peterson.

"Elias, there is disagreement as to whether the Resonex machine can work," Mike said. "Would you be willing to go and evaluate it?"

Mike and the chair of radiology, Martin Donner, sent me to Sunnyvale, California, south of Stanford, to look at the machine.

After arriving at Resonex at 8 a.m., I met Bill Brody. There was no time to waste, as I had a return flight to catch that afternoon. While I waited to see the machine, I asked Bill technical questions about it. He answered them. He explained the physics. He explained Resonex's history and its investors. Time was ticking away, and I still hadn't seen the machine.

Unbeknownst to me, after six months of running flawlessly, that morning, their MRI machine had stopped working. While they secretly tried to fix the problem by pulling the giant machine apart, Bill stalled for time.

"Elias, it's 10:30 in the morning, but it's actually 1:30 East Coast time, and there's a wonderful Chinese restaurant called Mings, just up in Palo Alto. Why don't we have some lunch, then we'll come back and see the machine when it's ready to be presented?"

After a delicious, early lunch, we returned. Secretly, Bill wasn't even sure if the machine was ready to work.

Thankfully, it was. I tested it and explored the software. It was years ahead of the software of other scanners. I was amazed. Hopkins needed this machine.

I took the redeye back to Baltimore. After returning, I told Mike we should purchase the Resonex machine. We met with Ron Peterson. Mike made a presentation. I expressed my support for the project and predicted that it would bring in a large number of research grants.

The problem was that the price of the Resonex machine (and associated costs) would be expensive. To complicate matters, Francis Scott Key was in a difficult financial spot. Ron Peterson had been hired to fix a hospital that was in total disarray. His discretionary fund was limited, and his needs were large. Would he really bet his money on new technology like the Resonex machine?

Ron looked at Mike and then looked at me. "If you guys stand by it and take responsibility for making it a success, I'll put my discretionary money towards it."

I was blown away. It was a gutsy move. I would always have a deep admiration for Ron.

His decision to bring in the Resonex machine would ultimately pay off, and it was a lesson in the value of taking risks. That's what great leadership is often about. It's about having the guts to take a chance—not a blind chance but a calculated one that can yield game-changing results.

The deal for the Resonex machine was supported by the radiology department chair, Martin Donner. In contrast, many radiology faculty were aghast. One of them said that working with cardiologists was worse than working with communists.

"They're our enemies, Elias. Don't you understand? They're going to eat your turf."

Despite faculty opposition, the deal happened, creating a relationship between Hopkins and Resonex through Mike Weisfeldt and Bill Brody.

For this new project, I started working with Ed Shapiro, who was now a cardiologist. Ed had been my guide during the radiology elective portion of my training at Hopkins in the 1970s. I was also happy to be working with Jim Weiss.

We all met every week at Francis Scott Key, discussing how we would advance our MRI project. It was a team of cardiologists, radiologists, and engineers. Mike Weisfeldt was there, and Bill Brody came from time to time, bringing even more ideas to the table. Bill had an exceptional mind, and it was a pleasure to work with him.

We needed to find a way to measure the contractions and mechanics of the heart by putting a marker on it. Rather than doing surgery and putting in a visible marker, I proposed that we could do it with a radio signal. We could put a radio frequency tag on the heart muscle itself and then image the heart as it was contracting.

"I don't know if it'll work, but it's a brilliant idea," said Bill Brody, who asked a Resonex engineer, David Parish, to help develop the software to implement the radio frequency tagging idea. David and I succeeded in our efforts and shared a patent for the breakthrough.

Meanwhile, conflicts with my MRI codirector persisted. Some faculty took her side, while others took mine. I tried to keep focused on my work, yet issues and tension remained.

I didn't know how to handle the situation. Maybe I was too forceful. This kind of forcefulness backfired by making the situation unworkable. Pushing too hard can be far worse than not pushing at all. My experience taught me a lesson in the value of soft but strong diplomacy, which I'd use in future conflicts.

Eventually, I decided that I'd had enough. I began looking for other jobs. I had options. I visited the chair, Martin Donner.

"Martin, this isn't working. I'm sorry, but I'd like to leave."

To my surprise, Martin didn't push back. "Yeah, Elias, I think this might be the right decision. Why don't you submit your resignation?"

I left his office, believing my time with Hopkins was over. Yet I didn't realize what was going on behind the scenes.

Exploring New Directions 11

I put in my resignation. It wasn't an easy decision. I had little savings, and I needed my salary. To pay the bills, I might have to accept a new job that wasn't ideal.

The lesson I learned here is the importance of having a financial cushion, or "getaway money." It gives you time to find the right opportunity. It also allows you to walk away more easily from a current job if circumstances take a bad turn, such as an ethical issue or a volatile disagreement. If you are not financially able to leave your job within 24 hours, you are in a vulnerable position.

With my last day at Hopkins approaching, I informed Mike Weisfeldt about my resignation.

"I can't tell you why, but don't resign," he said, withholding something significant.

What was he hiding? He wouldn't say. Regardless, my mind was made up. I was leaving.

That weekend, Bill Brody called me. He also told me not to resign.

"Why?" I asked.

"I'm going to be the next radiology chair, and I don't want you to go. You'll be a key member of my department."

The news caught me completely off guard. I knew that Dean Ross had been looking for a replacement for Martin Donner, who'd reached his retirement age. Yet unbeknownst to me, Ross had chosen Bill. It was all confidential.

The prospect of working under a brilliant physician-scientist like Bill Brody was enough to entice me to stay, as was his promise to work on fixing the codirector situation I was in. I'd expressed that I wanted to be a sole director of something.

Bill became chair, and eventually, my MRI codirector left for unrelated reasons. I was named director of the division in 1988.

We attracted fellows from all over the world. We built a successful division with terrific teamwork, and I evolved into a better leader. Yet my support among the faculty was not unanimous. I had unwittingly made enemies who felt threatened by my advancement and did not like my entrepreneurial bent. Academic politics could be difficult.

I became more conscious of my colleagues' intentions, of reading and better understanding what they were going through. The perception of reality was going to be different from individual to individual, even if based on the same set of facts. With this in mind, I became more patient, putting more care into what I said and how I said it.

Empathy and interpersonal skills are key ingredients of leadership. The growth I was undergoing here would be essential down the road, as I would step into positions of greater authority that demanded it.

While leading the MRI division, I became more aware of my flaws. Sometimes I could be blinded by my temper. Sometimes I could be too direct. I made changes to remedy these problems. Here, I observed that self-awareness was a fundamental precursor to personal growth.

～

The cardiac MRI tagging yielded a large multiyear research grant. The finances aided my lab, and with Bill Brody's help, in 1988, we brought on the brilliant Elliot McVeigh, a Canadian who had recently completed a PhD in medical biophysics. Elliot loved the idea of working on cardiac MRI. He had a soft, kind personality. He was always thoughtful and optimistic. Elliot wasn't just a brilliant scientist. He was also a great human being, and our research thrived because of it. Luck and care in recruiting the right talent would be a priority for us going forward, as it should be for any leader.

In time, MRI grew to become an important division at Hopkins, especially in terms of NIH grant funding, the currency of the realm. A biomedical imaging division was created in the Department of Biomedical Engineering. The division was led by Elliot. He trained outstanding graduate students who came to the MRI division in the hospital and worked on both basic and applied research topics.

Next, we approached the Department of Mechanical Engineering and the Department of Electrical Engineering, getting them to work on cardiac tagging with us. We were creating an ecosystem that was multidisciplinary and that encouraged scientists to have joint appointments. Soon, we were one of the top groups in cardiovascular imaging in the world. At this point, we were flying.

The diversity of our open, multidisciplinary approach was like a magic formula. It was a revolutionary shift from the siloed way things had been done. In 1990, an article about our lab was published in *Science*, praising it as being an example of the labs of the future. It was a new, multidisciplinary way of conducting research, eliminating artificial barriers between physical and biological scientific disciplines. It would eventually become common practice.

Our lab attracted numerous fellows and brilliant students, such as Mike Atalay, Scott Reeder, and Claire Tempany, and foreign physician-scientists, such as Christian Herold, Mario Muto, and my cousin, Alain Rahmouni (and many others), all of whom succeeded in ushering this open approach to innovation in medical imaging.

~

As I continued with my research, I also again stepped into the world of entrepreneurship. This second entrepreneurial adventure came from an idea that, like the multidisciplinary lab, combined many things into one.

In radiology, every modality was done separately. There was a CT center, an MRI center, an ultrasound center, and so on, all separated from each other. This created duplication in computing, technicians, and space.

I envisioned an integrated imaging center with different modalities combined into one location and with supercomputers capable of reconstructing and displaying images in real time. In this center, if MRI, CT, and ultrasound machines were linked through an optical network and connected to high-speed digital printers, one could increase productivity and reduce costs tremendously while serving many more patients.

I told Bill Brody that this was the way we should reorganize the radiology department. He was receptive, but many faculty weren't. Everybody wanted to keep their turf and keep things separate. Unfortunately, I wasn't going to be able to do this at Hopkins.

"Look," Bill Brody said to me. "If you want to do an outside venture, I'm for it."

At the time, Hopkins didn't favor entrepreneurial activities, yet that didn't stop Bill from granting me a leave of absence, with the understanding that I had to return. Moving forward, I chose to do my new venture in Virginia so that I wouldn't compete with Hopkins. Virginia was also favorable for another reason. In that state, a certificate of public need had been required to open an MRI center. Yet the legislation that mandated this had expired. There was a window of time before it would be renewed. I would open my center during this window.

At this point, I'd already contacted my good friend Bruce Holbrook and told him my idea. He was all for it. I also brought on Bill Drury, who was still managing CIRS. He would assist us with getting the operation up and running.

In terms of the machinery needed, due to my good relationship with GE, they agreed to lease the MRI and CT scanning equipment without a personal guarantee. Kodak could provide a digital printer on trial. The computer for image reconstruction from Silicon Graphics would be pricey, however.

The imaging center we would create would be called Advanced Medical Imaging Institute (AMII). At the time, hospitals were where imaging was carried out. The costs—and the prices faced by patients—could be hefty. We aimed to prove that outpatient imaging, which was more affordable, was the future. We also aimed to prove that an integrated model had value.

Bill Drury helped find a location for building the imaging center that was central to the Hampton Roads metropolitan area. I wanted to construct a state-of-the-art, truly first-class outpatient radiology facility. With our innovative design, we needed only 4,000 square feet or so, less than a third of the size most might've expected.

I went to my old radiology group at EVMS, led by Fred Stitik, and offered them the opportunity to provide the services for the center once it was built. They were interested.

Meanwhile, I worked on getting the financing together. I didn't have the money for construction and other start-up costs. Despite an ongoing crisis in the savings and loan industry, I was able to take out a loan and mortgage my house. Nadia helped by pledging her jewelry. After all this, I was still about $700,000 short.

I almost pulled the plug on the project. Bruce stopped me. He was confident that we could succeed.

"No, no, no. Let's go see your bank," he insisted. "You've been a good client. Let's see what we can work out."

We talked to them. They refused to help. We went to another bank. They also said no. Unfortunately, we were in a nationwide savings and loan crisis.

We eventually approached Dominion Bank. Bruce knew a man there named Paul Keister. Paul liked our project, yet his boss was hesitant about giving us the loan.

I came down to Norfolk to meet with them. We went out to the Harbor Club, a nice, waterside venue. It was Paul, his boss, Bruce, and me. Bruce and I explained everything about the project. I said it would break even in nine months. Yet they still weren't sure if they wanted to do the deal.

"You guys don't know who you're talking to," Bruce said, frustrated, trying to make it simple for the bankers to understand.

"What do you mean?" Paul and his boss asked.

"Look across the table. You see Elias? He's the Michael Jordan of radiology. If he's telling you they're going to break even in nine months, I guarantee you they'll break even before that. And if he does get in trouble, with his reputation, he can leave Hopkins and go anywhere in the country and make half a million bucks a year as a radiologist."

They gave me the loan, though not without many guarantees from my end. I agreed to the terms. What was the worst that could happen? I might fail and need to find a job and rebuild.

With the money, we now had the means to make AMII happen. Unfortunately, at the last minute, Fred and my old radiology group backed out of running the center. It wasn't their fault. The hospitals they were working with saw AMII as competition. They didn't want Fred and his group to work with us.

For now, I had to run the center myself. I explained the situation to Bill Brody, who responded kindly. I would work a day or two a week at Hopkins to maintain my research grants and team while spending the rest of my time with AMII. It would be a lot of driving, yet it wouldn't be forever.

"It's not going to take two years," I assured Bill Brody. "I'll launch this thing. I'll find a solution. I'll recruit some radiologists, train them, and I'll get some technicians."

I did all the above. The center opened. The demand was through the roof. It didn't take us nine months to break even. It happened far faster than that. Within seven days, we had more volume than we'd planned on for the first three months. As a result, the bank loan was repaid in full within a year.

Success triggered opposition. The local hospitals, which had been gouging people on MRIs, felt threatened. The legislation mandating that a certificate of public need was required to open an MRI center had long kept the hospitals' pricey monopoly of this imaging intact. Yet the expiration of this legislation had given AMII a chance to crack the monopoly wide open.

To strike back at AMII, the hospitals pressured their doctors to not send patients to the center. In response, we put together a marketing team.

We quickly learned that the doctors were not the decision-makers for ordering imaging. It was their nurses and assistants. We concentrated our marketing on them. It was successful.

A key lesson here is that the important decision-makers in an organization might not be those highest on the totem pole. If you're working with a business, you need to identify who the actual tactical decision-makers are so that you can build relationships with them.

~

During the AMII venture, it also became clear to me that doctors were no longer the ones deciding where their patients could be diagnosed. It was the increasingly powerful hospital systems, allergic to less pricey independent competition. This reality has only strengthened and evolved into the present, with monopolistic health systems formed by acquiring most hospitals in an area (including buying formerly independent physician groups) emerging as a counterforce to the few consolidated insurance company giants that have purchased and control thousands of physician practices.

~

AMII continued to prosper. We offered superior service and prices. We were sticklers for performance, and the output of the center remained high.

For head of operations, I'd brought in Keith Penn-Jones, a radiology technician colleague and friend who I'd worked with at Hopkins. I'd also hired my former CT technologist from EVMS. Like Keith, she was a wonderful, dedicated employee. She and Keith were invaluable at AMII.

The story of Keith Penn-Jones touched me deeply. An African American who overcame an impoverished upbringing in East Baltimore, I admired Keith's will, resolve, and intelligence.

Hopkins had a program where they took promising teenagers from the neighborhood school, Dunbar High School, and gave them summer internships. Keith, who grew up nearby, was awarded one of these internships, working in the nuclear medicine division under the head technician, Jim Langan.

In 1980, Keith began pursuing a certificate in nuclear medicine technology at Hopkins, which he received after two years. As a technologist, Keith quickly rose through the ranks. He applied to work in MRI to learn this new technology. He was hardworking, intelligent, and ambitious. Eventually, I had to name a chief technologist for MRI. I interviewed the candidates and liked Keith the most. He was the best, though some who were prejudiced might have disagreed.

As chief technologist and then later as head of operations at AMII, Keith did a fantastic job. He would further his education, obtaining a bachelor of science in business and a master's in business administration.

Keith was a gifted individual, born into circumstances that hid his potential from the world. All he needed was a chance. He was given that opportunity by Johns Hopkins, and he soared, rising through his own hard work and self-will.

I wonder how many other gifted men and women are hidden beneath poverty and poor circumstances? How much stronger would our society be if we gave them a chance regardless of the color of their skin?

It's important not to judge someone based on the color of their skin, their gender, their sexual orientation, their religion, or other factors. As an immigrant from a Muslim, Algerian background, I know what it's like to be judged based on appearance rather than substance. Prejudice of this sort is unjust and idiotic. It's the antithesis of what America truly stands for.

~

With the success of AMII ongoing, while still on partial leave from Hopkins, I eventually began a third entrepreneurial adventure.

At Hopkins, I obtained a grant to use high-resolution MRI to detect breast cancer. Through this advanced imaging, one could see the tiniest of lesions. This was helpful given that breast cancer needed to be detected early so that its spread could be prevented. Yet how could one verify whether these tiny lesions were cancerous?

A surgeon could perform a lumpectomy, removing a sizable amount of breast tissue. Yet afterward, the surgeon couldn't find the tiny lesions they'd taken out. Similarly, when I scanned the sliced-off tissue with MRI, I couldn't find the lesions either.

Another option was to do a needle biopsy. A doctor used a large needle, sticking the breast multiple times until they finally thought they'd sampled a lesion. Unfortunately, this procedure could not be done in an MRI machine. Perhaps if the biopsy was image-guided in real time and used a better needle, it could be more effective.

One day, Bruce Holbrook and I were having lunch. I mentioned the inadequate needle that was used for breast biopsies.

"Elias, why don't you invent a better needle?"

I took a napkin and started drawing the plans for one. Meanwhile, Bruce was drinking iced tea through a straw. He looked at the straw, expression shifting as he flipped it out. He'd come up with an idea.

"Why don't you just suck it out?"

Bruce was on to something. His words fueled my imagination. I developed the idea further.

Later, I met with Bill Brody. I proposed a breast biopsy method that was image-guided and used a needle with a vacuum that would suck up the tissue of interest after a single, much less invasive puncture. What I was proposing could be best achieved through mammography.

Bill thought it was a good idea. We went to see the inventor and entrepreneur, Dr. Tom Fogarty. Fogarty liked the concept and felt it could be done. Engineers were brought in.

Our team fully fleshed out the basic idea for the device and put together the technology. I was credited as one of the inventors. The contributions of those around me helped perfect the device into a feat of masterful engineering. The vacuum-assisted needle could efficiently produce high-quality tissue samples that yielded accurate diagnoses, all through just a single puncture.

Our invention was a success. It was widely adopted. Eventually, Biopsys Medical would be purchased by Johnson & Johnson in 1997. Our biopsy needle would be in continual use for decades, right into the present, affecting the biopsies of millions of women.

~

Prior to founding Biopsys, I returned to Hopkins full-time in 1992. Fred Stitik and his group were finally able to provide radiology services for AMII, and the institute was eventually purchased by a larger diagnostic imaging company.

During the period after my return to Hopkins and before Fred and his group went to work at AMII, Dr. Alexander Chako (who we'd recruited from Hopkins) continued to read films for the institute, often working late into the night. A superb radiologist, he played a key role in AMII's success and was a high-energy teammate.

Lessons learned from my early years with CIRS were reinforced through my AMII experiences. Not giving up, even when it seemed like the banks wouldn't lend the money, was key. If you have a great idea, you've got to be willing to fight for it. You've got to be willing to hear "no" a thousand times. Always ask yourself, what is the worst that could happen? If it's manageable, take the plunge.

You've also got to stay malleable in terms of how you go about trying to get what you want. If an obstacle arises and you fail to surmount it one way, look for a new path forward. Think through the process and come up with a solution. Nothing is impossible.

AMII's customer-focused culture and model was also an essential ingredient to the company's success. Like with CIRS, we had worked to understand what the customer wanted. In the end, it paid off.

~

Some of the radiology faculty at Hopkins felt my entrepreneurial activity was unbecoming for a Hopkins faculty member. They were philosophically against it. At the time, Hopkins wasn't open to entrepreneurship like Stanford or MIT. Bill Brody was trying to change this. Allowing entrepreneurship could bring immense benefits to an institution.

At Hopkins, some colleagues were also upset by the fact that I was promoted to full professor as soon as I returned. They didn't think it was fair after my leave of absence. They didn't know that my promotion had been approved prior to the leave.

Meanwhile, I received two chair offers, both from less reputable institutions than Hopkins. I explored them, as they gave me the opportunity to be in charge and not have to deal with the current conflicts in my department.

Soon, more prominent chair offers started to arrive. The University of Michigan invited me to visit their department. Nadia came along. I interviewed with Michigan's chair of the Department of Internal Medicine, Tadataka "Tachi" Yamada.

Later, Nadia and I were taken out to dinner. Michigan was trying hard to woo us.

"You know, madame," one of the Michigan faculty members, who knew my wife was half French, said, "the good thing about being here is that you can easily go to Detroit and fly directly to Paris."

During the car ride back to the hotel, Nadia gave me some valuable advice: "If somebody is telling you the best thing about a job is how fast you can get out of town, you shouldn't take that job."

I decided Michigan wasn't the right fit. Unfortunately, during the process, some colleagues from Hopkins who were against me called Michigan to try to spread hurtful rumors about me. These colleagues claimed I was dishonest. They criticized my entrepreneurship. Michigan backed off as a result. To Tachi Yamada's credit, he was in favor of me regardless of what my colleagues had said.

"So, he's an entrepreneurial guy, what's wrong with that? Are these Hopkins people crazy?"

~

Bill Brody was one of the smartest people I knew, and he realized that Hopkins medicine was in danger because of the fundamental conflict between the hospital and the medical school. The former increasingly favored patient care and financial performance over research and teaching. The medical school was led by a dean and the hospital by a president, and neither had full power over the other, leading to gridlock. As had been the case for my co-directorships, this coequality yielded problems. The trustees at Hopkins had created a board for the hospital and a board for the university, and they'd never really said who was to be a tiebreaker between the two.

Bill tried to intervene to solve the conflict. He wanted to put the hospital under the medical school in terms of authority. His idea was the right one. If we did the opposite and let the hospital lead, we would lose our connection to the innovative research engine that had made Hopkins what it was.

The status quo remained, however, and Bill ended up leaving his position as chair to become provost of the University of Minnesota. Bill's departure left me with a sense of loss. It also opened the door for a battle to see who would become the new chair.

The jockeying for succession started. The search committee was chaired by the head of orthopedics. They were not going to interview internal candidates until they had seen external candidates first. In the meantime, a member of the faculty would be the acting chair.

I didn't think I would ever be chair. I wasn't politically savvy, and I thought there was a glass ceiling for immigrant foreign medical graduates. I wasn't a graduate from Harvard, Penn, or Yale. On top of that, I was an entrepreneur. Meanwhile, Nadia, who was always my strongest supporter, believed I would become chair.

"I'm going to make you a bet," she said. "I bet that you'll become chair. And if I'm right, you'll figure out a way for me to build the house of my dreams."

I readily agreed to the bet, thinking I would never have to pay it.

The search progressed. The committee looked at outside candidates, followed by internal ones. The head of neuroradiology, Nick Bryan, was favored. He was kind and smart as hell. I would gladly have worked for him. Nasty, completely false rumors about his management style started to swirl, however, as ambitious and less qualified rivals sniped at him, hurting his chances.

At the time, the search committee hadn't called me. A colleague told me I wasn't even being considered. Meanwhile, I'd received calls from Yale regarding their chair opening. Would I consider being a candidate?

At Yale, I interviewed on the search committee's last meeting day. I was tentatively offered the position, subject to submitting acceptable plans and budget requests for the job by Tuesday, which was only a few days away.

The news of the Yale offer reached Hopkins. Soon, the head of the search committee at Hopkins called me and gave me surprising news.

"Elias, you have a chance to become chair here. We didn't call you yet because we didn't want you to come out too early, as it would've given time for the snipers to snipe at you."

I learned the committee was currently considering another candidate and would make a decision on Thursday. Meanwhile, Yale needed an answer by Tuesday.

I received a call from Yale. They told me I was asking for too large of a budget to run their radiology department. I pushed back, sticking with my request. I also learned they had been hearing negative rumors about me from Hopkins colleagues who spoke to faculty members at Yale. Yale was now reconsidering the job offer they had made to me.

Soon enough, I received yet another call from Yale. They'd offered the position to a physician who was rumored to be Hopkins's top candidate for chair. I was flabbergasted, yet it wouldn't be the last call I received. The head of the search committee at Hopkins called me again.

"Good news, Elias. Our top candidate decided to become chair at Yale. That opens the interview process for you."

The ensuing interview was thorough. I was now the favorite candidate at Hopkins. The sniping started, arising primarily from faculty members who had ambitions to become chair themselves and their friends.

Despite all the sniping, the search committee informed the current dean, Michael Johns, that they preferred me provided that the allegations against me were cleared. After a full investigation, the dean's office found no substance to any of it. The dean told the search committee that I should be appointed the next chair.

They did so unanimously. In November 1995, I was officially named.

Hopkins was looking toward the future by selecting a younger candidate with a different vision than more senior and established faculty. This kind of forward-minded hiring is essential when building out the executive team of any organization. Although, to be clear, it's not about hiring youth. It's about finding leaders of any age with the right mindset, energy, and fresh ideas.

One day, after I'd already been chosen as chair, I asked Dean Johns, "How did you make the decision to support me? Frankly, with all the noise and sniping, I may have backed off if I were you."

"Elias, you have something written on your forehead that nobody can deny."

"What's that?"

"Leadership." He pointed to his forehead and said, "You have leadership, and that's what we want you to do for this job."

The Challenges of Managed Care and Becoming a National Cancer Institute Adviser   12

I received a call from Rick Klausner's assistant. I didn't know Rick personally, though I knew he was a successful, brilliant scientist and the new director of the National Cancer Institute (NCI), of the NIH.

I learned through Rick's assistant that he wanted me to help develop a strategic imaging sciences plan for the NCI. I declined, as I was busy at Hopkins. Also, I was familiar with the bureaucracy at the NCI and the number of ideas that were proposed and never put into action.

A few days later, I received another call from Rick Klausner's office. This time, it was Rick himself. He was articulate, gregarious, and funny.

"Elias, you're the first person in my new job to turn me down for something important. What is that? Nobody turns down the NCI director."

I laughed, enjoying his sense of humor. As we conversed, Rick asserted the value of developing a strategic imaging sciences plan. He was looking for something visionary.

"How can you turn me down? It'll be carte blanche, Elias."

"Listen, I'll do it under two conditions. First, whatever plan we recommend, good or bad, you can say yes or no, but you cannot say maybe. I'm tired of working for the NIH bureaucracy. I always end up working on reports that end up in drawers and nothing happens."

My second condition was that if Rick wanted me to chair this effort, I would pick the members of the committee. I didn't want a homogeneous, one-size-fits-all group. I also didn't want to just cover clinical imaging. I wanted to cover molecular and cellular imaging. Imaging from molecule to man. Rick agreed. We moved forward.

Bill Kaelin, who would receive the Nobel Prize in Physiology or Medicine in 2019, was among those who joined our outstanding, leading-edge, multidisciplinary committee, which included cell biologists, brilliant physicists like Paul Bottomley, and others.

Working with the committee was a terrific experience. We had stimulating, fruitful discussions. We touched on how imaging was more than just acquiring images and reading them. It was extracting biological information noninvasively and modifying biology with tags and radioactive molecules. One could see a future in which single-cell analysis and single-molecule analysis would be done with imaging. As we formulated a strategic imaging sciences plan, an exceptionally bright Hopkins radiology resident (who was my first faculty hire after I became radiology chair), Marty Pomper, provided invaluable help.

Ultimately, the plan we produced was a success. Rick loved it. Rather than saying no or maybe, he said yes! He wanted to financially support the entire cell and molecular imaging program we proposed by putting many millions of dollars into it. Rick was a breath of fresh air at the NCI.

He invited me to serve on the NCI's Board of Scientific Advisors. I would do so from 1998 to 2002. The position would give me a window into the good, the bad, and the ugly of the NIH, into the fundamental mechanisms and real drivers of the agency.

~

Back at Hopkins, the conflict between the hospital and the medical school persisted, as coequality yielded problems. In the background, managed care had made tremendous inroads into controlling the practice and pricing of medicine. Insurance companies were excluding Hopkins for many services. They were negotiating prices for reimbursement that were often below cost and thus punitive. The financial situation at Hopkins was deteriorating rapidly. The faculty was in turmoil.

The chairs were also in turmoil. The Hopkins system made the chair of each department at the medical school also the chief of service for that department in the hospital. As chair, one had two bosses: the president of the hospital and the dean of the medical school. As I've said before, a person cannot serve two masters, nor can two masters lead one organization.

The conflict between the dean and hospital president affected life for the chairs, who wanted a reshaping of the Hopkins structure. Some chairs wanted the medical school, which valued teaching and research, to be preeminent. Others stood with the hospital, which valued patient services and financial performance.

After I was named incoming chair, I studied the situation, trying to formulate the right solution. Ultimately, I didn't see Hopkins evolving away from its traditional value of combining research, teaching, and patient care. I favored making the medical school preeminent while letting the hospital compete as effectively as possible under a unified board.

Meanwhile, the Hopkins Board of Trustees was undecided. Michael Bloomberg, who would selflessly donate billions to his alma mater, bettering Hopkins with his extraordinary generosity and philanthropy, was chair. He was frequently on campus trying to unravel the ongoing crisis. Philanthropists and businessmen George Bunting (chair of the Board of Trustees for the Johns Hopkins Hospital and the Johns Hopkins Health System) and Morris Offit (past chair of the university's Board of Trustees) were also actively trying to help solve the crisis. Their efforts were sincere and diligent.

As the crisis swirled, I tended to the reality of being an incoming radiology chair. In academic tradition, an incoming chair negotiated a package of resources, known as a dowry, for the benefit of their department. For my dowry, I needed resources as well as new modes of functioning and policies.

The radiology department wasn't allowed to expand beyond the hospital. Meanwhile, Hopkins hospital had expanded into limited outpatient services, which included radiology, in Baltimore City. The institution had given the radiology outpatient contract to outstanding former faculty member Nagi Khouri.

By being trapped in the hospital, the Hopkins radiology department was a victim of managed care companies. Some excluded Hopkins radiology because it was too expensive, a by-product of the hospital charging a hefty price for services. By being excluded, the radiology department lost patients. In a nonprofit academic center, one had to sustain their programs by obtaining revenues from the faculty practice.

If Hopkins wanted me to formally become radiology chair, they needed to give me permission to expand beyond the campus. Through experience, I knew that outpatient radiology was the future. I also requested funds for my department, though I knew the financially struggling medical school couldn't give me enough. Thus, I needed to be given the freedom to be entrepreneurial (within the limits of conflicts of interest rules).

I wouldn't formally accept the job of chair until I'd completed the dowry negotiation, yet this negotiation wasn't moving forward. I couldn't secure a meeting with both the hospital president and the medical school dean sitting with me and discussing a three-way deal. The relationship between them was too unhealthy.

Years later, a colleague, chair of anesthesiology and critical care medicine, Ed Miller, would recall, "It got so bad that the board was thinking of making them put their two desks together so they would talk to each other."[1]

The other chairs and I were collectively called in by the Board of Trustees and Nobel laureate Dr. Dan Nathans, who was the interim university president. The board and Dan Nathans understood that some of us were in favor of the hospital, while others supported the medical school. They wanted to hear our opinions. The chair of the Department of Orthopedic Surgery, Richard Stauffer, spoke up.

"I've been in this business for 23 years. I've never seen it so bad. This is not going anywhere without your intervention. We need a resolution. This is not sustainable."

I looked at the president, Dan Nathans, and asked, "Can I speak?"

"Go ahead."

"I'm not even a chair yet. I've been in this job for 23 days, and I've never seen a situation as bad as this."

The room erupted with laughter. Although my words sparked humor, they reinforced what Richard Stauffer had said. We were both experiencing a crisis. The meeting ended without a workable solution.

Later, Dan Nathans called me. He wanted to know how the situation was affecting me.

"I can't get anybody to listen and really think about the future of my department under my leadership and have a serious discussion. It's all nice conversations followed by no next step."

Dan intervened on my behalf. He had the dean and the hospital president each appoint someone with signature authority to negotiate. Rich Grossi, senior associate dean for finance and administration, and Ron Peterson, the Hopkins health system's chief operating officer, were chosen.[2]

I gave them a white paper that explained my plans for the department. Rich and Ron agreed to my key requests, including the freedom to create radiology practices outside of campus. After our agreement was approved and signed, I officially accepted the job of chair, knowing I had the means to make an impact.

Being chair wasn't about the prestige. I wanted to achieve something rather than just pad my résumé. No job should be taken for the prestige alone.

I was present as Dean Michael Johns informed the radiology faculty that I was now officially the department chair.

"You have to reunite behind your new leader. I know some of you had other opinions about who should be in charge, but this is the direction the institution decided on, and based on what Elias negotiated, I can tell you, this department is going to go in the right direction."

Afterward, Dean Johns and I talked in private. I learned he would be leaving Hopkins by the summer. I would lose a key ally. Dean Johns was liked by the faculty and had stood by us. How would we fare without him? I went home, wondering what I'd gotten myself into. The crisis was deepening.

~

Early in my tenure, I met with the man who'd been managing the radiology department's finances.

"Elias, we're in trouble."

"What do you mean? We're one of the richest departments."

"The billing system at the faculty practice isn't operating properly."

For the faculty practice, collecting money from surgeries and other big-ticket items was deemed more worthwhile than bringing in $10 from a chest X-ray. As a result, the radiology department was not a priority and was losing around (as best as I can remember) $500,000 a month. I would have to use part of my dowry to cover salaries. Meanwhile, the radiology faculty hadn't been given a raise for the past few years.

I visited the managers running the faculty practice for the medical school. It was a mess.

I later relayed this reality to the outgoing dean, Michael Johns, and the interim dean, Ed Miller. Ed, then the chair of anesthesiology and critical care medicine, was handsome, white-haired, charismatic, kind, and diplomatic.

"Do you know how much money you're losing per year with the current system at the faculty practice?" I asked. "Relative to your budget, you will be in a deficit of $15 million this year."

"Do us a favor," they said. "We want you to meet with the managers of the faculty practice weekly. You'll be part of the executive group there."

I did so. I pushed for internal reform of the practice's billing system and a renegotiation of insurance contracts.

Soon, I was informed by Ed Miller and Michael Johns that I would be made executive vice dean and president of the faculty practice. It would be a heavy lift to do this new job on top of running the radiology department, and my reputation would be on the line. Additionally, the added responsibility meant that I would no longer have time to practice medicine and see patients, the most enjoyable part of my job. I liked working with physicians and researchers who needed my expertise. I enjoyed solving diagnostic riddles.

Yet I needed to take on this new role to help Hopkins and my department, in that order. I agreed to start my new job under the condition that I be given the authority to properly execute my duties. I wanted full authority over the contracting of doctors and to be chair of the board of the faculty practice. I wanted real power to make real changes, and I wanted to report only to the deans.

It's always important to make sure your authority in a job matches its responsibilities. If this isn't the case, you are being set up for failure.

~

All the department chairs collectively formed the board of the faculty practice, for which I was now, suddenly, chair, just a few months after becoming head of radiology. Typically, a chair of radiology didn't have a prominent role in the larger institution, particularly when compared to the more clinical and sizable departments of medicine or surgery. Over time, however, this changed. There were more radiologists like Bill Brody, me, and others who assumed major roles in their institutions. We understood the system and had large-scale management experience, which became essential in academic medical centers.

Radiology was now a major component of the hospital. The department had well over a thousand employees and was unbelievably complex and difficult to manage. I could not be successful as a radiology chair by simply going into my office every day and looking at whether the X-rays were read well and on time. For me to succeed, I had to be involved in the ecosystem of the school, hospital, and marketplace.

As executive vice dean and president of the faculty practice, I collectively met with the managers of all the departments at the faculty practice. Most lacked the needed experience. The practice had to be run as a professional operation with key performance indicators, benchmarks, and milestones. We needed new leadership.

I informed the board of the faculty practice about three new hires I wished to make, a qualified trio of candidates. The chairs researched my choices. There was a false, slanderous report received about one of the candidates.

The chair who had received this report complained to Ed Miller. This chair didn't respect my authority because I was only the head of radiology rather than a more traditionally prominent division of medicine.

Confident in my choices, I told Ed Miller, "Do you want him [the chair who had complained] to run this thing, or me?"

"I gave you the job, Elias. So, you just have to control this, and I'm going to have them sign on to your candidate's appointment. And if they don't, you know what to do."

"What do you want me to do?"

"You got to bring them to the woodshed."

Ed Miller turned out to be a terrific, strong leader who would have a great tenure at Hopkins. The two of us soon met with the disgruntled chair.

"I hear he's no good," the chair said of one of my candidates. "And appointing him should be the decision of the major departments, not the chair of radiology, with all due respect."

Ed shot back, "For whatever reason, this institution is in trouble, and you're a big part of that. Right? So, if it's in trouble, you have responsibilities. And oh, by the way, if you think surgery is special and the other departments are not, let me dissuade you from that notion. We're all equal. And we are all team players. Are you on board or not?"

The chair eventually conceded that Ed was right. "It's true we're in trouble. And, Elias, if appointing this candidate is what you believe we should do, I'll support you. I'm loyal to the institution above all else."

I was impressed by the chair's words. In putting the institution above himself, he was sacrificing for a greater good. In the present, society could benefit from more of this behavior. The pendulum has swung too far in favor of self-interest, to the point where institutions we depend on suffer greatly.

Another takeaway from this meeting was Ed Miller's brave leadership. He wasn't afraid to do the right thing, no matter how difficult. Dominating one's fears is a key part of leadership.

The new administrative team for the faculty practice arrived. We worked for roughly six months reorganizing our processes and brought in a new computer system. We moved forward with renegotiating unfavorable managed care contracts.

"Guys, we're Johns Hopkins," I stated. "We're not some fly-by-night operation. They give us the same contracts that they give far lesser hospitals. . . . People are going to come to Hopkins because of the quality of what we do."

I believed we should try to prove to at least one insurance company that what they were doing to us was destructive to them as well. At the time, we were negotiating with a major one.

"If you don't have Hopkins in your network, your business will suffer," I insisted to them.

"Dr. Zerhouni, with all due respect, you don't really get it, do you? The world has changed. Yeah, doctors decided everything in 1980. But now, managed care companies are here to control your crazy costs."

The insurance company pushed me to sign a bad deal. I refused. Our hospital went berserk, not wanting to lose patients. Yet I believed the insurance company would come back to the negotiating table. Without us in their network, they would lose countless patients.

Sure enough, after about two months, the insurance company came back. Their enrollment was crashing. We negotiated a new, favorable contract. It wouldn't be our last victory.

With better contracts and management, the faculty practice was turned around in about a year. In the meantime, Hopkins was looking for a new university president. I went to Minnesota to visit my former colleague Bill Brody and discovered some interesting news.

"Hopkins approached me about the position. What do you think?"

Bill was the right candidate for the job. Regarding the hospital and medical school conflict, he understood both sides of the equation, and he knew the solution, which was creating a dean/CEO position and putting the hospital under the medical school in terms of authority.

In 1996, Bill was chosen as president of the university. His tenure would be transformative and successful. In the end, years later, he'd leave Hopkins far stronger than he'd found it.

The trustees restructured the Hopkins medical school and hospital to have a dean/CEO who was dean of the medical school and CEO of the newly created Johns Hopkins Medicine, which was overseen by one board. The head of the hospital now reported to the dean/CEO, who was Ed Miller. The problem of coequality was resolved. The Hopkins medical school and hospital, both among the world's best, were now unified.

Pulse Management   13

At Hopkins, I was executive vice dean, president of the faculty practice, and chair of the radiology department. While working many jobs simultaneously, I wondered about how to manage so many tasks. Unconsciously, I developed an approach whereby I would involve myself fully for about three to four months in an issue, grasp it and define an approach, and then hire the people who could implement this approach. Regarding those whom I hired, I delegated them full authority and responsibility, asking them to come to me only if there was a problem they could not address themselves. Over time, I came to appreciate the efficiency of this approach, which I eventually named "pulse management."

The best analogy is that of a plate spinner with multiple plates spinning on multiple sticks at the same time. The plate spinner sets each plate in motion and then fixes them if they start to wobble. Plate spinners successfully spin four or five plates at the same time provided that the plates are well balanced (or, in my case, if the right leaders have been chosen to oversee each responsibility).

In essence, my approach was to set an enterprise in motion, delegate responsibilities to selected leaders, and then shift my attention to whatever other project needed my help, providing a pulse of energy to put it back on track. After putting this project back on track, I then moved on to the next issue that arose. Pulse management gave me time and energy to take on increasingly large amounts of responsibility and grow stronger teams. Meanwhile, a hefty workload and schedule prevented me from falling into the trap of micromanagement.

~

Soon enough, I would add a fourth job at Hopkins with the creation of a company called American Radiology Services (ARS). ARS would be born from the freedom I was given as radiology chair to create practices outside of campus. Prior to ARS, the local outpatient radiology community laughed at Hopkins. They thought we were bureaucratic, slow, and not truly service oriented. They aimed to create a belt of imaging centers around us and eat our lunch.

To respond, we had to expand into outpatient radiology services immediately. I enlisted the help of Bruce Holbrook as well as his intelligent and capable brother-in-law, Carey Kriz, who was working in the radiology department as the executive director of the Center for Biomedical Visualization. We assessed the situation and began moving forward.

The problem was that, as radiology chair, I had the freedom to do what I wanted, yet I couldn't truly utilize this autonomy. Nagi Khouri had been given the rights for Hopkins outpatient radiology in Baltimore. He had a center in Greenspring. I couldn't break his contract. Yet Nagi's contract was causing problems for him as well. It prohibited him from joining competing radiology groups, putting him at a disadvantage.

At a Radiological Society of North America meeting in Chicago, I took Bruce Holbrook aside and told him to speak to Nagi. I wanted Bruce to try to buy Nagi's center and get the rights back to outpatient imaging. I knew Bruce could get the deal done quickly and quietly.

Bruce and Nagi went for a cup of coffee. During their meeting, they agreed on a purchase price and employment guarantees, subject to my approval. Bruce and Nagi had no paper, so they wrote down the terms on a napkin, which they brought to me. Nagi and I signed the napkin, and the deal was done.

We built a full-service imaging center at Nagi's Greenspring location following the AMII model. Next, we acquired an imaging center positioned along the Baltimore beltway. Visible to traffic, the center had great signage, yet it was struggling financially. The center wasn't part of an outpatient group and was a victim of managed care. I promised the doctor running the center that he wouldn't have to cover its losses and would be employed by Hopkins.

We upgraded the center's equipment and purchased a huge neon sign advertising Johns Hopkins Imaging. Day or night, you couldn't miss it. The sign woke up our competition.

Yet rather than focusing only on battling my competition, I envisioned a company, ARS, that could merge competing practices together so that they could combat managed care companies, which were now consolidated into mini monopolies. If I could assemble a group of radiologists who would make up one-third of the market (a threshold that wouldn't violate antitrust law), with Hopkins as the only academic partner, I could challenge managed care rather than being a victim of it. Bruce, Carey, Ted Segal, and Joanne Pollack (the latter two being attorneys) helped me design the strategy we'd use to bring ARS to life.

Carey, at times accompanied by Ted, went knocking on doors, speaking with the heads of rival radiology practices and explaining the advantages of us coming together. For our team, it was round-the-clock, grueling work. For Carey, the phone was ringing at all hours, day and night. From start to finish, building ARS would be a massive undertaking.

Bruce convinced a major bank to give ARS a nonrecourse loan so that the company could acquire all the practice equipment of the various radiologists who wanted to join. The radiologists had personally guaranteed their existing equipment loans. The loan Bruce obtained eliminated the doctors' financial exposure, which many of them had been worried about as managed care slashed their revenues.

Ultimately, we had 18 hospitals and 33 imaging centers interested in joining. This geographically strategic assemblage included much of the hospital and outpatient radiology around the Baltimore beltway in addition to contracts in southern Maryland.

With the financing in place, the next task was convincing the multitude of lawyers representing all parties that this transaction made sense. It was tedious work. In one meeting, Bruce counted 20 or more lawyers in the room. Eventually, the deal went through.

Insurance companies were shocked that a group of doctors, with Hopkins as the academic partner, had come together. It was a cultural shift they never saw coming.

Consolidation came with challenges, however. To obtain an accurate understanding of the company's financial state and future, we had to slice and dice loads of data from different practices and assemble a strong financial department. We discovered that we were losing money and needed to rethink our model.

We conceived a business plan that led to the closing of old, poorly located centers and upgrading others so that they'd have top-of-the-line, AMII-caliber equipment. Of the 33 imaging centers, we closed 15 and upgraded the 18 that remained.

Consolidating and centralizing advanced radiology modalities would be one of the main drivers in ARS's turnaround. Meanwhile, centralized scheduling and improved practice efficiency would also play a role, giving patients a better experience and fueling positive word-of-mouth reviews. Yet another key to ARS's success would be contract renegotiations with insurance companies.

In managing and shaping the company, we used frontline data from our staff. We sent a questionnaire to every one of them. Among other questions, we asked what they felt was or was not working in the company. What would they change about operations if they could? Additionally, our management team interviewed every staff member, using their feedback as a basis for making changes. The staff felt empowered. Including them in our company evaluation process became a consistent point of culture in ARS.

In a broader sense, getting feedback is a helpful tool for anyone in a position of leadership in an organization. You need data to help shape your decisions. It's also helpful to have such data in hand when forming and pushing forward initiatives. It allows you to build with collective desires and needs in mind.

$$\sim$$

One of the reasons ARS succeeded was the leadership of CEO Bob Carfagno. It isn't enough to have a business plan. You need a leader who can execute. Bob was this and more. He was indispensable. I remain grateful for all he did.

Among the other incredible colleagues who helped ARS succeed, Keith Penn-Jones (who had been integral to AMII's success) also played a key role, ascending to the position of vice president of operations and business development.

ARS was a new kind of radiology practice, a distributed network practice with electronic communications and extreme efficiency. Images would be shared between centers through the internet so that they would go to the best specialist. Films were often sent to Hopkins, where they were read by my faculty. This brought additional money into the department. We could now invest in new faculty members and rebuild the nuclear medicine division.

Colleagues saw that our proactive, outward push had worked. It became a model for other departments at Hopkins to follow.

Proactivity is a key takeaway from the ARS experience. If we'd sat back and waited for managed care and rival imaging groups to tighten the noose around Hopkins, it could've been devastating. If you're in a crisis, a new strategy is key, yet so is swift, decisive action.

Eventually, ARS was purchased. A colleague of Carey Kriz named Jonathan Gurgler, a former surgeon from Harvard who was working for a private equity fund, helped arrange a substantial buyout. This buyout generously compensated the physicians involved in ARS. It also yielded many millions in funding for Hopkins and my department while maintaining the reach of the latter in a community that valued our services.

In looking back on the ARS journey, Bruce felt we couldn't have succeeded without the experience gained from building and running AMII as well as the early on-the-ground efforts of those like Carey Kriz and Ted Segal. With AMII, many in Hopkins radiology had attacked me for being entrepreneurial. Yet it was this entrepreneurial pursuit that yielded knowledge and experience that would serve Hopkins in its hour of need.

~

As I continued to balance responsibilities and roles at Hopkins, the Nobel laureate and former NIH director, Harold Varmus, who was president and CEO of Memorial Sloan Kettering (MSK) Cancer Center in New York, asked me (at the recommendation of Hopkins's Dr. Marty Abeloff) to review his radiology department. I came to know Harold more closely and ultimately provided a review he valued, which led to major changes under his leadership and that of Dr. Hedi Hricak, the chair of the department.

I also became an ad hoc participant in some sessions of the scientific advisory board at MSK regarding diagnostic radiology as well as radiation oncology and nuclear medicine. Being in these advisory sessions was eye-opening. I was in the company of extraordinary minds, sitting next to molecular neuroscientist and biologist Richard Axel, who would win a Nobel Prize in 2004 for his discoveries related to the olfactory system. I witnessed interactions between leaders at the top of molecular biology and oncology. I came to understand the fundamental dynamics of these fields as well as the process that Harold used to successfully lead MSK.

While working with a former NIH director, I also witnessed a change within the NIH that I'd supported: the creation of the newly born National Institute of Bio-Imaging and Bioengineering (NIBIB). My entire career, I'd witnessed in frustration as the main NIH institutes were generally unwilling to embrace emerging technologies unless they directly applied to a disease relevant to their scope of research. This problem had been extraordinarily limiting for radiologists, who couldn't obtain the funding they needed, resulting in useful emerging technologies being neglected. The NIBIB helped solve this issue.

My efforts in supporting the NIBIB's creation had included lobbying Congress alongside other scientists and defying those at the NIH who opposed the project. The grassroots effort to create the NIBIB had taken many years and the persistence and dedication of countless individuals. Through this battle, I'd learned much about government and the NIH. I didn't realize it, but it was yet another set of experiences preparing me to eventually become director.

~

One day, while out of town, I received a call from several department chairs at Hopkins. They wanted me to become vice dean of research, an area that needed a turnaround. They recommended me to our dean/CEO, Ed Miller. Ed came up with the idea of having Bill Baumgartner, who was on the board of the faculty practice, take my place as president of it so that I could shift into overseeing research.

Given how much I enjoyed my current research-related activities, I gladly took on this new role. Meanwhile, dealing with the faculty practice had become too routine for me. I craved new challenges. The brilliant head of basic sciences, Dr. Thomas Kelly (who would, in a career filled with impactful contributions to science and medicine, direct the Sloan Kettering Institute from 2002 to 2013), was quite supportive of my becoming vice dean of research. I liked his no-nonsense approach to issues. We became good friends and colleagues.

My new role came with challenges. Top-notch scientists had to be recruited. New areas of science needed to be explored. New buildings and labs needed to be built.

The departments were fighting over research space. Employing a rational approach to the problem, we conducted an inventory of all the space, noting what each department had. Meanwhile, we determined the research grant dollars per square foot that each department was contributing.

Our map of data illuminated major imbalances. Some departments that had underperformed in research funding were getting too much space. Others that were thriving were getting too little.

We brought together the department chairs and other key players and presented the data. It was curated and reliable. Rather than telling my colleagues my conclusions, I was helping them reach them on their own. They could double-check the data.

We had an open, no-holds-barred discussion about everyone's concerns and drove to a solution. We aimed for a quantitative approach to the management of research space and ended up with a system that fairly allocated and reallocated it. The allocation system opened the door to the creation of new research buildings on campus by convincing the board that we needed more space to grow. The system also paved the way for an eventual biotech park and entrepreneurial expansion around the campus.

Meanwhile, I supported the idea of institutes without walls to create multidisciplinary structures where scientists would mix and match regardless of their departmental affiliation or discipline. We'd had success with my multidisciplinary lab, and I wanted to use this approach to better the overall state of research at Hopkins. New frontiers of medicine could not be reached without a synergy of disciplines.

Accordingly, the school created an interdepartmental institute for genomic medicine as well as one for basic sciences. With the help of an extraordinarily generous donation from Michael Bloomberg (who, at the time, donated anonymously), we also founded an institute for cell engineering, creating synergy between engineering and biology.

The changes we made helped Hopkins receive more NIH funding. Overall, my time supervising and understanding basic research at Hopkins was fulfilling, and it gave me an experience that was useful when I went to the NIH, as I better understood both the clinical and the basic research worlds.

When trying to reach a consensus and get colleagues on board with a vision, presenting accurate data, having an open discussion, and driving to a solution are a trifecta that can equal success. In my experience, colleagues will reach a consensus in the majority of cases when reliable and transparent information is shared.

Another lesson here is the value of a quantitative approach to solving management issues. Time and again, I used this approach to solve issues in different medical departments and businesses. I also used it in science, as I brought quantitative approaches to imaging biology.

~

Hopkins had earned major victories, yet it was still facing major challenges. As executive vice dean, all the deans told me their problems. One day, I asked the associate dean for admissions, Jim Weiss, what his number one issue was.

"When we offer a position to a prospective medical student, who has also received an offer from Harvard, in roughly 75 percent of cases, they go to Harvard. They don't come to Hopkins. I'm really concerned about it because that wasn't always the case. Before it was 50/50. Every year, I'm seeing more students not wanting to come to Hopkins."

Exit interviews revealed that a key reason was related to the dangerous neighborhoods surrounding the campus. If our facilities were not attractive and the campus was not safe, it would be hard to keep recruiting the best medical students, residents, scientists, and others.

To help remedy the problem, we came up with the idea of creating a biotech park that would reshape the part of campus that was most dangerous and difficult to manage, an area of abandoned houses. I wanted to push this project forward to help the local community as well as Hopkins. I was met with internal opposition. My colleagues wanted to help the neighborhood but were worried we'd be accused of gentrification.

Not everyone was against the idea, however. The distinguished Hopkins neuroscientist Solomon Snyder suggested I speak with the Abell Foundation (which was "committed to improving health, economic, and educational outcomes in Baltimore City so that all people can thrive").[1] Sol introduced me to the foundation's president, Bob Embry.

I requested money for a feasibility study for a biotech park project that would replace the north side of campus. Bob contacted a consultant who then conducted research and informed us that the neighborhood had to be completely destroyed.

"There's nothing left to save except the historical monuments. If you put in a biotech park, housing, and a biotechnology magnet school for the community to train the local students, you may have a chance. You also need to cover relocation for the families who live there."

The first phase would cost (to my recollection) around $25 million. I went back to Hopkins and was met with more resistance. Colleagues wanted to help the local community, but there was concern that there would be a political storm if we did the project. To avoid this outcome, I needed to better understand the politics of Baltimore.

Amelia Arria, who was on the faculty at the Johns Hopkins School of Public Health, recommended I meet with an African American leader in the faith-based community, Charles Gordon. Charles ran a faith-based ministry for those who had been incarcerated and reintegrated into society.

I sat down with Charles, and he explained the politics of Baltimore.

"You'll have a lot of naysayers, but at the end of the day, if you get Delegate Pete Rawlings, who is head of appropriations, Mayor Martin O'Malley, and Senator Nathaniel McFadden, those three, they'll hold the key for you."

One of the Hopkins trustees was close to Mayor O'Malley (who later became governor and ran for president) and was able to get me an appointment with him. O'Malley and I met, and he loved the project. He convinced Delegate Rawlings to get on board.

Meanwhile, Senator McFadden was opposed. Eventually, O'Malley had me and the senator come to his office. I explained the project to McFadden. He wanted his community to have a return on it.

"It's not gentrification, I know. But we have to have our share," McFadden insisted.

After some discussion, McFadden suggested I talk to the community, including top business leaders.

We would have, as Delegate Rawlings called it, "a meeting of everybody." The attendees included Rawlings, McFadden, politicians from East Baltimore, individuals sent by the mayor, and members of the African American business community, among others. I was in the room with around 25 people who wanted to understand what the project was about and to decide if they were going to support it.

I explained the project to the room, showing them a slide presentation. I was bombarded with questions: How much can you guarantee us if we do the development? Who's going to do the building? Who's going to get the contracts? There was strong opposition, fed in part by suspicions regarding Hopkins's intentions. The desires of special interest groups were also feeding the resistance in the room.

Eventually, my frustration reached a boiling point. I'd brought a big binder with me that had transported slides for my presentation. I slapped the binder closed, almost theatrically. The room calmed down. I expressed my frustration and articulated that, as important as this project was, I had many other duties to fulfill for Hopkins. I stood up to leave and thanked them all for coming.

"Doctor, sit down," Delegate Rawlings said. "Please sit down."

There was silence. I could tell Rawlings was in charge. He was a Sphinx-like figure who didn't talk often. To quote the *Baltimore Sun*, Rawlings "had the mind of a trained mathematician and the fearlessness of a man certain of his convictions."[2]

"I personally like the project," Rawlings stated. "We have to find a way to make this happen."

After that, it was smooth sailing, and we would ultimately succeed in turning the biotech development project into a reality.

At Hopkins, Bill Brody, Ed Miller, Ron Peterson, Sally MacConnell, and myself would be among those who played a role in the project's ultimate success. To quote Greg Rienzi of the Hopkins *Gazette*, "The plan comes as a result of a unique partnership between the Mayor's Office, the state of Maryland, Johns Hopkins, the Historic East Baltimore Community Action Coalition and the communities of East Baltimore."[3]

Many parties were involved in making this project work. Like many accomplishments, it took a village to pull this one off. The $200 million, 80-acre development project would provide housing units, green space, jobs, and a biotech park that could include as many as 50 companies.[4] I would leave Hopkins just when the deal closed.

"There will not be another project like this in most of our lifetimes," said Democratic representative and extraordinary civil rights leader Elijah Cummings (who would serve in 13 terms of Congress). "This is an historic moment in a wonderful place called East Baltimore."[5]

⁓

During these years at Hopkins, while juggling many duties, I stayed committed to my role as radiology chair. When I started, internally, there was plenty of conflict between faculty members. Morale wasn't always high.

To help, we reinforced our leadership team and created a new culture. I kept the wise Bob Gaylor in his role as vice chair. He was an administrative guru who understood the business of radiology and how to make a department efficient. I asked Stan Siegelman to be a vice chair as well. Stan was universally respected. He was incredibly productive, a good human being, and a great mentor. I needed to send a message that contributing to the department earned one recognition. By promoting Stan, I did.

"Elias, when you came to this place, you could barely speak English. Now here I am reporting to you as your vice chair."

Stan had recently lost his wife, Doris, to cancer. Nadia and I had been close to her. I wanted Stan to have more responsibilities at work to distract him from his grief. He was depressed, and being a swimmer like me, we trained together a few times in the pool.

Stan and I were longtime friends. His mentorship and help had been crucial. A Jewish American doctor had enabled my Arab American success story. This is the greatness of the United States, a country that challenges bigotry and, at its best, rewards merit regardless of race, gender, or creed.

⁓

With Stan and Bob Gayler, I had vice chairs I could delegate responsibilities to. This gave me time to handle issues in the department that needed my direct involvement. I examined our divisions and observed the balance between clinical work, teaching, and research. I wanted my department to be research driven.

Yet traditional radiology faculty were heavily involved in clinical work and teaching while not putting as much time into research. I built a cadre of young radiologists interested in doing the latter. I encouraged the most creative ones to stick around. Winning the war for talent was a key to success.

I had to identify those who were exceptional. For example, I promoted Elliot McVeigh to head of MRI research, appointed the talented David Blumke as the clinical director in the MRI division, and eventually appointed the remarkably smart neuroradiologist Norm Beauchamp as vice chair for clinical operations.

Meanwhile, I opened the financial books to the division directors. Doing so allowed each director to see the budget for their respective division and if that division was making or losing money. They hadn't had access to such data before. I felt it would help them properly drive their divisions. Ultimately, it made the department more productive.

Giving employees an objective report card can help you get the best out of them. Rather than simply telling employees what you want them to do or how you want them to improve, show them through reliable data. Here again, I stress the importance of making accurate data available when it comes to getting others on board with a vision.

Through no fault of their own, my division directors didn't have enough business management experience. They'd built their careers in an era where few academics ventured into entrepreneurship. We worked to provide them with needed education. For example, we organized lectures about budgeting and profit and loss management.

Dr. Cathy DeAngelis and Toby Gordon, ScD, helped create a business of medicine certificate at the medical school. I sent my best faculty to attend the program, taught by experts.

Meanwhile, we applied the same strategy in the medical school that we had in my department. We opened the financial books to the chairs, giving them valuable data. The improvements were substantial.

~

In the radiology department, the division of nuclear medicine was revitalized. We'd generated the income needed to upgrade our equipment, which made it possible to recruit a top-notch new director. Following a lengthy pursuit, Richard Wahl, whom I'd met through my work at the NCI, was brought on. He gave the division a real boost.

I placed my former resident, Marty Pomper, who was now a professor, into nuclear medicine, encouraging him to pursue molecular imaging. Not surprisingly, Marty excelled. He would one day be the director of nuclear medicine and molecular imaging, a promotion well deserved.

By the end of my tenure as chair, I would leave a hefty financial reserve, partially because of the ARS deal. The department was sitting on more resources than when I started. It had gained in the national rankings for research and clinical care.

~

Although I was often busy with work, at home, I managed to be there in the critical moments for my children, as did Nadia. Throughout the years, we'd supported their education and found ways to have fun with them. For example, we'd attended plenty of sporting events, including Orioles and Ravens games (to this day, we remain huge Ravens fans). We'd also imparted life lessons and taught our children about their Algerian, Muslim heritage.

I wanted to teach them everything I could. I also wanted to spend more time with them, yet work was unrelenting. I would regret all the hours I missed with them.

Thankfully, Nadia was there in my absence. As a mother, she was a tigress, always ready to protect our children. Their education and welfare were her number one priority. She was an extraordinary mother while also balancing a career of her own as a pediatric endocrinologist. I've said it before, and I'll say it again: I couldn't have achieved what I have without her.

~

My son, Will, whose intelligence was always off the charts, attended Harvard for his undergraduate studies. He went on to study at Harvard Law School. He'd always wanted to be a lawyer. It would be exciting to see him live out his dream.

Yasmin went from being a delightful girl to a delightful young woman. She had a strong character while always knowing how to navigate situations without hurting feelings. She was simultaneously laid-back and ambitious. Her life path would eventually take her into medicine, as she studied at Hopkins and became a surgeon, now at City of Hope in Los Angeles.

Meanwhile, Adam was in his teens. He was brimming with creativity, passion, and empathy. He would grow to become an extraordinary artist, not unlike my granduncle, whose beautiful music and poetry had shaped the Moorish-Andalusian culture of Nedroma, my place of birth.

~

Life became financially comfortable for my family as a result of the Biopsys venture. The success of this venture paved the way for the creation of Nadia's dream house. Before I'd been chosen as chair, Nadia and I had agreed on a bet. If I became chair, I had to figure out a way for her to build the house of her dreams.

After I'd been chosen, Nadia looked at me and said, "I'm waiting."

We went looking for waterfront land to build on. We found it, about a half-hour drive from Hopkins. Nadia hired the construction team and designed every piece of the house, recruiting a young architect to help. It would be a spacious, contemporary home, with high ceilings and fantastic views of the water. I was glad I'd lost the bet.

~

By the end of 2001, after turbulent years fulfilling many roles at once, I wanted to return to my department full-time and take a breather. I wanted more regular hours and some quiet. Unbeknownst to me, I would soon be considered for the role of NIH director. My life would be transformed as I stepped onto the highest political stage of biomedical research.

THE NIH

III

The White House Is on the Line 14

"Dr. Z, the White House is on the line," my assistant said with a bewildered look of urgency.

It was December 2001, and we were in my office at Hopkins. On the other end of the line was an assistant to the head of the Presidential Personnel Office, Clay Johnson III. The assistant wanted to schedule a phone call with me and Johnson's deputy, Ed Moy.

Meanwhile, I'd recently been contacted by the NIH through Dr. Steve Katz, the director of the National Institute of Arthritis and Musculoskeletal and Skin Diseases (NIAMS), who was leading the search for the director of the newly created NIBIB. Steve had wanted me to be considered for the position. I'd declined, craving normal hours after having shouldered such a large workload at Hopkins.

Now, as I sat in my office, with Clay Johnson's assistant on the line, I wondered if Steve Katz had reached out to the White House to use them to persuade me about the NIBIB directorship. Assuming this was the case, I agreed to schedule a call with Ed Moy as a courtesy, with the firm intention of declining the White House's request.

During my eventual call with Ed, I received shocking news. He wanted to know if I would agree to be considered for the role of NIH director. Leading this colossus of an agency, with its 27 institutes and centers, was no small task and no small honor. While not having the public recognition of other government organizations, such as the FBI or the CIA, the NIH was essential to the health and well-being of all Americans. It was, to put it simply, "the nation's medical research agency."[1]

I requested time to consider the offer. I discussed it with Nadia. Bill Brody had given the White House my name. He felt I could succeed as director, though part of him wished I wouldn't get the job, as he didn't want Hopkins to lose me.

"It felt like giving away my right arm when I recommended you, but it's for the good of the country," Bill told me.

Putting country above self was admirable. Bill, like countless scientists outside of and within the NIH, had a sense of duty to society that guided his actions.

Although Bill Brody felt I'd succeed as director, I didn't have the traditional pedigree for the job. I wasn't known as a basic research scientist. I was a radiologist and a foreign medical graduate. I still felt there was a glass ceiling for how high I could rise. Being chosen for the job was a long shot.

And if I was chosen, following in the footsteps of the agency's last director, Nobel laureate Harold Varmus (who I'd gotten to know after he asked me to review his radiology department at MSK and whose legacy and accomplishments as NIH director had been extraordinary), wouldn't be easy. Meanwhile, the NIH was facing challenges. Its budget was on the path to being doubled soon, yet the agency needed a new strategy for the coming century. The entrenched bureaucracy and the troublesome tendency of institutes to jealously maintain their autonomy remained ongoing problems. Meanwhile, the NIH was also feeling the heat of the fiery political controversy regarding federal funding for embryonic stem cell research.

I was no stranger to stem cell research. At Hopkins, I'd helped create an institute for cell engineering. Embryonic stem cells had significant therapeutic potential to treat a number of cruel diseases, including Parkinson's and Alzheimer's. Yet the cells were obtained from deliberately destroyed human embryos, a reality that upset numerous religious conservatives, among others.

During the entire Clinton presidency, White House opposition ensured that no funding for stem cell research was ever granted by the NIH. This was why I'd had to raise funds from Mike Bloomberg to create an institute for cell engineering at Hopkins. We had needed private philanthropy to make up for a lack of federal funding.

In 2001, the landscape shifted. Going forward, research on the existing 78 embryonic stem cell lines could be supported by federal dollars. Yet, according to President Bush's announcement, these existing lines were the limit. It was a Solomonic decision, and though the president's policy was limiting and would ultimately not be enough, it was at least a step in the right direction that, for the first time, opened federal funding for this research field. Many scientists were furious about the limitations, however.

The overwhelmingly liberal scientific world, politically hostile to the Bush administration and its pro-life, antiabortion supporters, had made the issue of NIH leadership a political one. Many assumed a right-wing scientist would be chosen as the next director. In contrast, I was a registered, apolitical Independent. I was a politically naïve scientist, a dangerous thing to be in Washington.

～

To learn more about the job of NIH director, Bill Brody recommended I sit down with Hopkins trustee and retired ambassador Sol Linowitz. I met Sol at the Cosmos Club for lunch, a key hub for Washington power brokers. Sol, now well into his eighties, entered, cane in hand. He had a patrician demeanor, and he attracted the immediate attention of the staff. On our way to his chosen table, many saluted him.

We sat down, and Sol dispensed with niceties, immediately asking how he could be helpful. I confessed that I knew nothing about politics, government, or federal agencies. I wanted his views on why I should even consider the NIH directorship.

Sol smiled and said, "This may turn out to be the best and worst decision of your life."

NIH director was a highly visible political appointment, and these were times of vicious political conflict. If I became director, Sol told me I would lose my right to speak freely. He also had something to say about the thousands of employees I would oversee at NIH.

"Every one of them can and will create mischief that will end up being a nightmare for you. Every day you will be at the mercy of circumstances beyond your control. Your job will be to avoid being featured above the fold of the *Washington Post* in a scandal that could tarnish your reputation forever."

His words underscored the stakes and dangers of leading the NIH. I was opening myself up to a new world of threats.

Sol went on to say, "Your reputation is the single most important asset you have. Are you prepared to lose it? To risk it?"

Sol later told me to take the job of director not for its prestige but instead for what I believed the agency needed to do to improve and better serve the people. This was in line with my thinking. As I'd mentioned in chapter 12, one should never take a job simply for the prestige.

Next, Sol asked me what I would do if I were appointed director. I was still formulating my thoughts. My role on the NCI scientific advisory council had given me a window into the good, the bad, and the ugly at the NIH. I knew the agency needed change.

"Elias, any change you will want to make is bound to create negative reactions simply because you will be disturbing a myriad of special interests. On the other hand, all negative things aside, the responsibility of NIH director is a unique opportunity. I'd consider it seriously. It is a privilege few are offered."

Sol pointed out that one of the first things I had to do if I became director was figure out who could fire me and in what order. First was the president, who could do it in a millisecond. Therefore, it was essential I developed a strong rapport with him and his team. I needed to make sure that I had direct access to the president and that colleagues knew I had his confidence.

The NIH director also reported to the secretary of the Department of Health and Human Services (HHS). Therefore, I also had to find a way to work well with them. Finally, the powerful chairs of congressional committees could also fire me, though not as quickly as the president. I'd need to build relationships on both sides of the aisle.

～

Following my lunch with Sol, as I drove home, my mind was swirling with thoughts and scenarios, ranging from good to bad. Through working with former NIH director Harold Varmus at MSK, I'd learned about some aspects of the tribulations of being agency director.

Harold had told me that, during his tenure, he'd developed several areas of scientific emphasis he and the scientific community at large thought were key to progress. Yet the powerful institutes within the NIH, which received direct congressional appropriations, often ignored or slow-walked these recommendations. The institutes felt that the recommendations were outside of their authorized missions.

While the institutes did, at times, pursue objectives beyond the more basic boundaries of their missions and did, at times, collaborate with each other, the current structure of the NIH was, as many in the scientific community described, a confederacy rather than a federation. This situation was exacerbated by the director's lack of independent financial resources. The director had too little power, while the 27 institutes and centers had too much. Through their constituencies, which often used powerful lobbyists, they resisted more central coordination by the director. The NIH was like a hand with 27 strong fingers and no palm.

If Nobel laureate Harold Varmus, with all his prestige, connections, and pedigree, was limited in his influence over the NIH juggernaut, how would I, an immigrant with a modest pedigree from Algeria, in a field (imaging and biomedical engineering) not typically considered as important or exciting as molecular biology, move the needle, so to speak? I was already on a good career path at Hopkins, and as I mulled over all the risks that went along with the NIH directorship, I wondered why I hadn't already called back Ed Moy and declined.

The answer was that Nadia had never stopped believing in me. I always felt as if I was both an insider and an outsider within American academic medicine. I dreaded the glass ceiling rumored to stifle the career of foreign medical graduates. Yet Nadia gave me confidence and courage. She pushed me to consider the opportunity of NIH director and to overcome my fears.

"It is part of your destiny. Live it and think about what it would mean for your children and all the immigrants who are working hard to contribute to this country like you. You can be an example for many who feel excluded," she insisted.

Her "yes, you can" speech led me to call the White House back to start the process. I was throwing my hat into the ring, though I wasn't fully convinced I would accept the job if it were offered. Part of me was still on the fence.

～

At the beginning of January, I met with Ed Moy. He was friendly and professional. He insisted on total confidentiality for the process of my being considered as director. The White House had done discreet inquiries about me and were encouraged by what they'd heard. They would soon do a thorough background check.

Ed informed me that the White House wanted an agent of change for the NIH. The administration had committed to continue the doubling of the NIH budget, yet both the White House and Congress weren't sure how these larger resources would be used for greater effect.

I told Ed the core issue at the NIH was the lack of larger strategic coordination between the powerful institutes and their constituencies. Additionally, science had evolved, creating gaps that no single institute could fill. The recent creation of the NIBIB had been successful, yet the NIH couldn't just keep adding institutes to fill every emerging gap. That would take years and lead to an even more complex, fragmented, and unwieldy agency. The NIH needed to find a better way to cover these gaps.

There was a better solution, and I wanted to find it. I argued to Ed that continuing the increase of the NIH budget could be a historic opportunity to attempt reform.

Ed was pleased with my comments. He asked me to develop my ideas further.

At the end of the meeting, Ed inquired about my family. I told him about Nadia, who was now running the International Adoption Clinic at Hopkins. Ed perked up, saying that he and his wife were in the process of adopting girls from China and would love to connect with the clinic. This helped establish the beginnings of a bond between Ed and me.

On the way out, I asked him why he hadn't brought up the fact that I was an immigrant. I was a Muslim in a post-9/11 world. Would that not be a problem for the administration?

"As long as you're a U.S. citizen in good standing and best fit for the job, the president will be happy to consider you. This is America."

As we parted, Ed mentioned they were looking at several other candidates. His job was to come up with a few for the president to choose from. Ed would work to set up a series of interviews for me, the first of which would be with Tommy Thompson, the secretary of HHS.

Days later, I went to HHS headquarters and met with Secretary Thompson. A national figure, he was charismatic and gregarious. We'd met once before during a short phone interaction on 9/11, when Ed Miller and I called him to determine what the Hopkins hospital needed to do on that terrible morning.

Now, as I met with Secretary Thompson in person, I could immediately tell he was not pleased that the White House had foisted me on him.

"My preferred candidate is Tony [Fauci]," he said point-blank.

I was taken aback by his bluntness, yet I realized he was directing his comments more to the White House liaison who had accompanied me. I learned later that Fauci, who knew the NIH inside and out, refused to assume the role of director if he had to relinquish the directorship of his own institute, the National Institute of Allergy and Infectious Diseases (NIAID). Tommy Thompson was fine with that, but the White House, apparently, would not agree to it.

After initial, harsh words, Thompson softened and asked me to tell him about how I proposed to change the NIH for the better. I told him that any agency reform had to be done soon while budgets were still increasing. We could create a common fund for the NIH director to use to address issues that the whole agency needed to deal with but that none of the institutes could tackle. This concept appealed to him.

"I much prefer Tony Fauci, but your ideas make some sense."

Thompson then brought up the topic of human embryonic stem cell research and where I stood on it. I told him that President Bush's decision to allow research on the existing cell lines was a reasonable step forward.

My meeting with Secretary Thompson ended, and in time, he reached out to Ed Miller at Hopkins. The two had developed a good rapport since 9/11, when Hopkins actively supported the national response. Ed gave me a glowing recommendation, trying to convince Thompson I was the right choice. Ed sensed that the secretary would be supportive of my nomination.

My successful meeting with Thompson, which started at rock bottom and ended with hope, shows what's possible when you face an interviewer, colleague, or adversary, who seems like they'd never say yes to you or your vision. There can be an instinct to shut down when met with this kind of opposition. Yet never underestimate the power of preparation and the words that come from it, to sway even the most ardent critic.

～

The process continued forward, and though things were supposed to be confidential, I discovered that nothing ever really was in Washington. I received a call from Ken Shine, the president of the Institute of Medicine, which I'd been elected to in 1999. He came to visit with me at Hopkins and told me that I was now in top consideration for NIH director.

The White House had contacted Ken to help vet the candidates. Ken was impressed with what I'd accomplished at Hopkins. Yet he knew that I had been a consultant to the White House in 1985 under President Reagan and assumed I was well-connected to the Republican Party. I told him I was a registered Independent with no political ties and my role under President Reagan had only been that of a medical consultant. This seemed to reassure Ken.

Next, he wanted, among other topics, to hear my views on human embryonic stem cell research. I repeated what I'd told Secretary Thompson. To me, the president's policy was a reasonable step forward that, for the first time, opened NIH funding for this research. Ultimately, my discussion with Ken went well.

Regarding sensitive issues such as stem cell research, at this point, I was well-equipped to discuss them. Part of my preparation had come from talking through the issues at length over the phone with my son, Will, who was finishing law school at Harvard, and was a politically astute adviser.

~

Momentum was accelerating in my favor. Meanwhile, I was still unsure about whether I would actually accept the directorship if it was offered.

I obtained Ed Moy's permission to speak confidentially with former NIH director Harold Varmus about the job. On a gray day in February, I took an Amtrak train up to New York City to meet Harold at the Harvard Club. As was usual for him, he arrived on his bike, casually dressed, wearing a helmet and a backpack.

Soon, Harold and I chatted in a dark, quiet corner of the club. He felt it would be wonderful if I was chosen as the next director. He thought I could do an excellent job. His words gave me confidence.

Harold spent the next five hours guiding me through the intricacies of the position. He noted how important the relationship with the White House and the secretary of HHS had been for him. It was also clear to him that building strong relationships with members of Congress would be essential to my success.

Harold educated me on the limitations of the director's influence over the institutes in addition to other issues within the NIH. Despite the issues he mentioned, Harold remained in admiration of the NIH, calling it the crown jewel of the federal government. I was both enthralled and intimidated by the scope of challenges and opportunities he described.

I was particularly concerned about whether the scientific community would accept me given my personal and scientific background. Harold brushed it off, saying that enough people knew me to reassure the community that I would serve with integrity and show appreciation for all fields of science.

Regarding the politically sensitive subject of human embryonic stem cells, Harold said the key was to stick to the science and avoid being drawn into the political debate. If I maintained my scientific integrity and acknowledged that the elected president was the final arbiter in making political decisions and I truthfully informed the administration and Congress about the science, I should be okay.

Due to the contested 2000 election, the mood in Washington was highly partisan. If nominated, I should expect a long and protracted confirmation process. Harold pointed out that his own confirmation occurred five months after being nominated. In the event I was chosen, I would likely have time to manage a proper transition out of Hopkins.

At the end of our long meeting, I crossed a tipping point. With his mastery of words, Harold had convinced me to take the plunge. If chosen, I'd say yes.

~

If I said yes, I'd be taking a huge pay cut. The financial cushion I had in place from my entrepreneurial ventures made me more comfortable with this reality. Other candidates who lacked my financial cushion might have been dissuaded, however. One of the drawbacks of becoming NIH director that has likely stopped some excellent candidates from being considered is that the job doesn't pay well enough to be competitive.

~

I traveled to Florida for a vacation with my family. Early one morning, while in my hotel room, a call came through from the White House. I spoke with Ed Moy, who informed me that my background check had gone well.

"Would you accept if the president selected you? I need an answer now," Ed said firmly.

I thought for a moment, and responded, "Of course."

The next day, I received yet another call from Ed.

"Clay and I met with 43 [their nickname for President Bush] this afternoon, and he really liked your story, and based on what you did at Hopkins, coming from Algeria, he felt you could do well at NIH, too. Congratulations."

I was elated. I thanked Ed and asked him to thank the president for me.

Ed described the necessary next steps, which included being cleared by the White House counsel and the FBI. The minutia of the clearance process was daunting. The FBI had to reach out to current and previous neighbors and employers in the United States and Algeria to ask about my character and behavior. Additionally, the White House counsel had an exhaustive questionnaire, looking for anything that could embarrass the president.

The process moved forward, and, to my surprise, I observed that the White House was working collaboratively with Senator Ted Kennedy's office. Was this an island of bipartisanship in Washington? It dawned on me that the transition from Hopkins to the NIH might be faster than I'd expected. Indeed, the process seemed to suddenly accelerate.

~

In the press, an article citing unnamed government sources revealed I was the likely nominee for NIH director. I was surprised, but friends told me the leak was likely orchestrated by the White House as a trial balloon to test the reactions of the relevant constituencies and discover any embarrassing facts about me the administration might have missed.

In response to the news, many Hopkins coworkers expressed both surprise and support. I became the topic of discussions. Colleagues reported receiving phone calls from their contacts at the NIH and elsewhere inquiring about me. Was I the right choice for director?

Beyond Hopkins, some scientific organizations spoke out in support of me. Influential organizations, such as Research!America (a nonprofit research advocacy alliance that championed science, discovery, and innovation to achieve better health for all),[2] were among the voices in favor. Over the years, I would come to better know Research!America's president and CEO, the brilliant Mary Woolley, who successfully led her foundation to become one of the most influential in Washington, supporting the NIH and other key agencies. I would learn a great deal from Mary about the best ways to communicate and advocate for one's mission.

Former congressman Paul Rodgers, Research!America's chair and a tireless advocate for bettering the health care of Americans, and former congressman John Edward Porter, a board member of Research!America whose dedication to advancing medical research was extraordinary, would strongly support my eventual nomination as director as well as my ensuing tenure. While they and others believed I could succeed as NIH director, there were some who felt I was unfit for the job. The then president of the Biotechnology Industry Organization, Carl Feldbaum, claimed I was on a mission to stop stem cell research, and he questioned my character. I was taken aback. Years later, Carl and I would serve on a board together, and he would apologize for having been misled, and we would become good friends. For now, however, he was a critic among others.

Thankfully, I had strong mentors and supporters, particularly among the radiology academic community. I also received plenty of support from other scientific communities. I greatly appreciated every person who stood by me. Of note was the reaction in my homeland, proud to see an Algerian-born scientist reach such a position.

~

In late March, President Bush would officially nominate me. In a post-9/11 world, where Islamophobia was rampant, his decision to appoint an Algerian Muslim immigrant to head the NIH was a bold move.

As a nominee, I wasn't going to try to score political points by distancing myself from my Muslim background. I wasn't going to sell out where I came from and betray the family and friends who had helped me throughout my life.

Life will challenge us with moments where it may seem easier to disavow parts of our identity rather than holding true to them. Yet self-betrayal comes at a high cost. What good is the greatest job in the world if you must change yourself in fundamental ways and betray those you love most to obtain it?

My nomination spoke volumes about the greatness of America. There is no other country in the world where an immigrant could develop such a career. Already, I felt like I owed more to America than America could ever owe to me.

On March 26, the president would announce my nomination. On the invite list for the White House event, I included colleagues from Hopkins as well as representatives of relevant scientific societies. I asked Harold Varmus to attend along with the NIH invitees. Family and friends were not forgotten. Nadia and my children, whose love and support continued to be invaluable, would attend, as would Bruce Holbrook, among other friends.

The day of the event to announce my nomination, I was to meet President Bush in the Oval Office beforehand. As I approached the office, walking the halls of the White House, I was accompanied by Secretary Thompson and the athletic, charming Dr. Richard Carmona (nominee for surgeon general), whom I had just met.[3]

On our way to the Oval Office, President Bush saluted Thompson with a friendly, "How are you Double T?"

The president gave nicknames to his staff, especially if he liked them. Over time, he took to calling me "Big E."

President Bush immediately put me and Richard at ease, showing us the Oval Office, including its famous portraits and sculptures. The president told me that he liked my personal story and what I'd done at Hopkins.

With his trademark squint and smile, Bush said, "Elias, look around this office. Enjoy it. If all goes well for you at NIH, this may be the first and last time you come here because if I have to call you back, it's usually not good news."

We laughed. I enjoyed the president's natural humor as well as his down-to-earth manners. I felt we would have a positive relationship.

Together, President Bush, Secretary Thompson, Richard Carmona, and I entered the East Room for the nomination event. My family was in the first row of the audience.

After opening remarks, President Bush introduced me and later recounted my arrival in America with my wife and only a few hundred dollars in my pocket.[4] I'd come a long way. As he continued his speech, the president urged Congress to approve an NIH budget increase of nearly $4 billion for 2003 (the agency's current budget was more than $23 billion).[5] It was reassuring to know I'd be serving under a president who was committed to helping the NIH.

At the podium, President Bush eventually declared, "Dr. Zerhouni shares my view that human life is precious, and should not be exploited or destroyed for the benefits of others."[6]

It didn't immediately dawn on me that the president was, with these words, signaling that I was fundamentally aligned with him on the issue of stem cell research. My son, Will, and Bruce Holbrook felt I was being jammed into a position that would be difficult to manage. In time, they would be proven right.

In a larger sense, I would have to learn to walk a political tightrope amidst the push and pull of right-wing groups and the scientific community.

Following the president's words, I read a short statement of thanks to him and the audience. In this moment, I felt such deep gratitude. Only in America could an immigrant be nominated to such a position.

"Mr. President, my family and I are touched by your nomination, because it says about our great country, what no other country can say about itself."[7]

Confirmation

15

Although I'd officially been nominated, I still needed to be confirmed by the Senate. I'd have to pass through another gauntlet of interviews. I thought the collective confirmation process would take months. Accordingly, I made relaxed plans for leaving Hopkins and taking a vacation.

Unfortunately, my vision of a leisurely exit from Hopkins didn't come to pass. Many didn't realize that Senator Ted Kennedy and President Bush had developed a good working relationship. Both men understood the enormous importance of having the role of NIH director filled promptly.

The legislative director of HHS, Scott Whitaker, was put in charge of shepherding me through the Senate confirmation process. I would have to meet with all the senators on the authorizing committee overseeing the NIH, known as the Health, Education, Labor, and Pensions (HELP) Committee, chaired by Senator Kennedy. Scott expected this would take months.

To his surprise, he was able to schedule a meeting with Senator Kennedy the next week. It would be my first confirmation interview. The process was already moving faster than expected.

When it came time for the meeting, I nervously entered Senator Kennedy's office and was asked by his staff to sit on the sofa. David Bowen, one of Kennedy's key aides, was present. Throughout the course of my eventual tenure as NIH director, David would be an example of a staffer whose public service was exemplary.

Senator Kennedy soon arrived for the meeting, entering with one of his famous Portuguese Water Dogs by his side. The senator was limping slightly and a little hunched because of previous back injuries. Yet his smile and jovial demeanor calmed my nerves.

We shook hands, and he recounted how he'd enjoyed visiting Morocco and Algeria in the 1950s. The Kennedys were quite popular in Algeria due to their stand for its independence.

"I never imagined I would one day be sitting with a Kennedy, talking about NIH."

The senator laughed. He looked at me with his expressive, blue eyes. "That's the American dream, Elias. I believe in it, and you're an example of it. This is what we are in this country. We welcome all immigrants of talent."

He asked me a few questions regarding my views about the NIH. I made general comments about the fact that science had evolved in a direction that was not necessarily aligned with the structure of the institutes. Something would have to be done to serve areas of science that were not specific to any one of them. He liked my answers.

Kennedy raised the issue of stem cell research. He said he would not question my beliefs on the matter and understood that I would have to follow the Bush administration's policies. Yet he wanted to be assured that I would faithfully inform Congress and the public of the scientific facts. I told him that I would.

The interview went on, and Kennedy and I seemed to get along well. During our conversation, his dog moved closer to me, and I petted him.

At the end of a meeting that lasted much longer than planned, Kennedy said, "My dog seems to like you, and I do, too. So, I will support you, and I hope we can have a hearing before the end of the month."

We were building the beginnings of a relationship that would be crucial during my tenure as director.

Scott Whitaker, pleased about the outcome of the meeting, told me, "Unless the Senate background check fails or a senator puts a hold on you for whatever reason, you'll be confirmed soon."

I'd find out later that Senator Kennedy had already done his due diligence on me prior to our meeting. He'd reached out to Ed Miller, among others. A true statesman, Senator Kennedy always did his homework.

More confirmation interviews came, including ones with the senators of my home state of Maryland, Democrats Barbara Mikulski and Paul Sarbanes. After meeting with Senator Sarbanes, with whom I got along well, I wondered if creating a personal connection on first encounters was a singular trait of successful politicians. I discovered later that it was indeed an essential part of being effective in Washington, particularly in Congress.

This kind of efficient relationship building can be beneficial in careers beyond Capitol Hill. It's important to establish a personal connection from a place of honesty, however. A lack of authenticity will backfire.

～

The meeting with Republican senator Arlen Specter from Pennsylvania, who asked to see me even though he was not on the confirmation committee, would not be so easy. Scott Whitaker and I met with the senator's staffers and chatted with them before Specter arrived. I felt no warmth. Something was bothering them.

When Senator Specter entered, after some formal introductions, he shifted gears. With a prosecutorial tone, he asked if I had to pass a litmus test on stem cell research for the White House to make me the nominee.

"No one asked me to pledge political allegiance of any kind or pass a litmus test. I stand for the science and leave the politics out of it and will do so at NIH."

After a few moments, Specter replied that he'd heard otherwise. As politely as I could, I told him he was misinformed. He squinted, expecting more from me perhaps. I stayed silent.

After a few moments, the senator said, "Okay, I believe you. But remember, I care deeply about the NIH. It's the crown jewel agency of the government. I'll be watching you."

Despite the tense nature of our initial interaction, over the subsequent years, Senator Specter and I would develop a mutually supportive and trusting relationship that would include his influential and effective staff (including Sudip Parikh, now the brilliant CEO of the American Association for the Advancement of Science), who became friends and supporters during my tenure. Specter's help would be crucial for my work at the NIH, and he was unwavering in his support for the agency and its budget, along with Iowa senator Tom Harkin. A champion for those with disabilities, Harkin was a public servant guided by empathy. He would make an admirable impact.

～

The date of the confirmation hearing would be April 30. This was less than two weeks away. Given the speed at which the confirmation process was unfolding, I was concerned about properly managing my transition out of Hopkins.

Meanwhile, my early confirmation interviews were followed by a flurry of meetings with the remaining, available members of the HELP Committee.

I observed remarkable bipartisan support for the NIH. My individual recollection of the fast-paced interviews would be blurry, except for a meeting with Democratic senator Paul Wellstone of Minnesota, who impressed me with his commitment to the cause of muscular dystrophy patients.

I also met the thoughtful, thorough, and intelligent Republican senator Judd Gregg, who expressed concern regarding the proper use of the new budget the NIH was receiving. He wasn't convinced it was being managed appropriately given the fragmented nature of the agency.

With the confirmation hearing fast approaching, Scott Whitaker encouraged me to start writing my testimony. To complicate matters, as was customary, prior to the confirmation hearing, I was not allowed to interact with the NIH.

To help prepare myself, I continued to discuss controversial issues, including stem cell research, at length with my son, Will. I also reviewed the testimonies of previous directors.

In my testimony, I wanted to stress the growing and necessary convergence of biomedical, physical, computational, and engineering sciences. Having a background in mathematics and physics and having applied both medical and physical science disciplines to my research, I knew how important it was for the future of science to open the NIH to the idea of supporting more than just biological researchers or physicians.

I would have to be specific about my vision and ideas regarding the NIH's future roles. Senators wanted to know more about how I would direct the NIH to use its rapidly increasing budget. Most were unsure how the agency should help address the country's health challenges.

Crystallizing and clearly communicating my approach while not appearing as having already made up my mind would be key. Balancing decisive clarity and openness of mind would be a challenge. If I were too vague and claimed I would study the issues further, I'd be seen as unprepared and weak. If I were too strong in my convictions, I'd be seen as presumptuous and arrogant. A subtle equilibrium must be achieved.

All the preparation in the world could not remove my anxiety about the hearing to come. Rather than succumbing to these fears, however, I worked to overcome them. Right or wrong, I would fully share my beliefs at the hearing.

I knew that the only way to succeed was to share my deeply held views with honesty. The quickest way to lose credibility would be to try to please constituencies at the expense of my own sincere beliefs.

It's not wise to assume a position of leadership under a different identity than one's own. It destroys the trust needed to convince others to join in

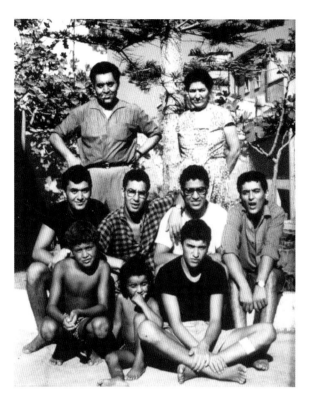

Taken in 1964 during my childhood in Algiers. Front row (left to right): Adnan, Moulay, and me. Second row (left to right): Boumediene, Moustafa, Chahid, and Ahmed. Third row: my father and mother. *Zerhouni family*

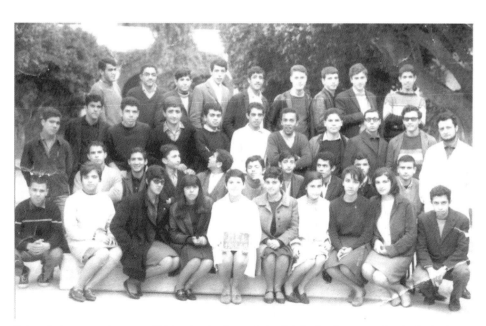

Taken during my senior year of high school at Lycee Emir Abdelkader. I was standing in the back row, second from the right, with my shoulder facing the camera. My lifelong friend Hachemi Oussalah was standing on my left. *Algiers Photographer*

A view of Algiers. *Alanphillips*

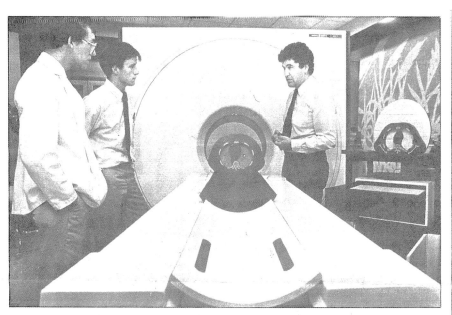

Model of human chest cavity helps determine whether lung spot is malignant
Zerhouni, right, shows his 'phantom simulator' to EVMS students Roger Watkins, left, and Scott Roberts

Device detects cancer without surgery

By ELLEN WHITFORD
Staff writer

It looks not unlike a child's puzzle: inch-thick rings made of epoxy resin that can fit inside each other, and a set of small white cylinders.

But the device, a piece of pioneering technology designed by a local doctor, is a diagnostic tool that could help eliminate millions of dollars in chest operations each year.

For patients like John Johnson, who had a solitary lung spot which his doctor thought was cancer, the device meant the difference between a procedure that cost a few hundred dollars and took less than two hours and a major operation that cost several thousand dollars and a month or two of recovery.

Two years ago, Johnson's family doctor discovered a spot on his right lung. And because the 55-year-old Norfolk airplane instrument mechanic smoked four packs of cigarettes a day, his doctor thought it might be cancer. When tests failed to show whether the spot was malignant, a surgeon decided to schedule him for surgery.

That's when Johnson's daughter, a sec-

retary in the radiology department at De Paul Hospital, suggested that he see Dr. Elias Zerhouni.

Using a CAT scanner, which X-rays a patient from a myriad of angles and produces images of the inside of the body, Zerhouni looked at the spot on Johnson's lung.

Then Zerhouni compared that picture with a scan made of the puzzle look-alike, a "phantom simulator." The phantom chemically simulates the human chest cavity. To the scanner, the phantom and Johnson's chest were identical. A small plastic nodule, containing calcium, simulated his lung spot.

The radiologist found that Johnson's spot was denser than the nodule, which meant that the spot contained a large amount of calcium. That, in turn, meant it was almost certainly benign; malignant tumors contain only small amounts of calcium.

Johnson, who was scheduled for surgery the following day at Norfolk General Hospital, instead checked out and went home.

— *Please turn to page D4, col.5*

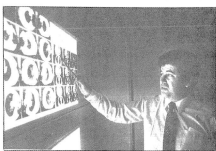

Staff photos by Tommy Price

Zerhouni checks images made by the CAT scanner

An excerpt of a 1984 article covering the Pulmonary Nodule Reference Phantom. *Ellen Whitford (article) and Tommy Price (photos), Virginian-Pilot/TCA*

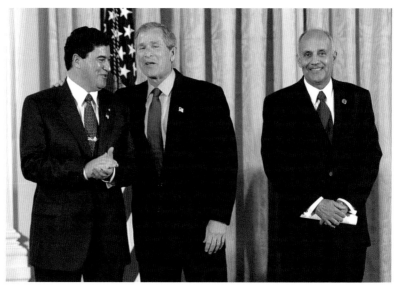

2002. Me (NIH director nominee), President Bush, and Richard Carmona (surgeon general nominee) stood in the White House East Room during Richard's and my nomination event. *Getty Images/Staff*

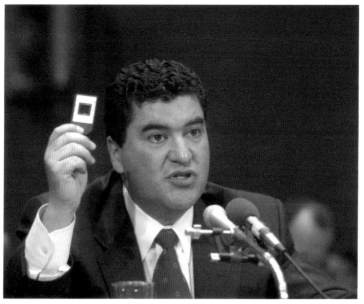

I held up a novel DNA chip, using it as a prop as I gave my testimony during the Senate confirmation hearing for my NIH directorship. I would be confirmed by a unanimous consent vote on May 2, 2002, becoming the fifteenth director of the NIH. *Public domain from U.S. Congress*

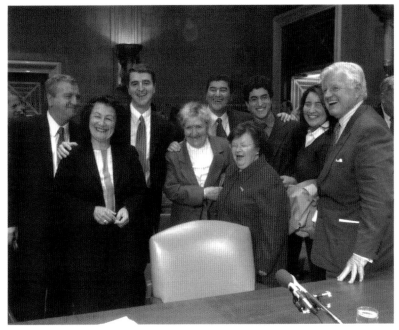

2002. From left to right: Hachemi Oussalah (my childhood friend), Nadia (my wife), Will (my son), my mother, me, Senator Barbara Mikulski, Adam (my son), Yasmin (my daughter), and Senator Ted Kennedy. We were gathered for the Senate confirmation hearing that would usher in my tenure as NIH director. *Public domain from U.S. Congress*

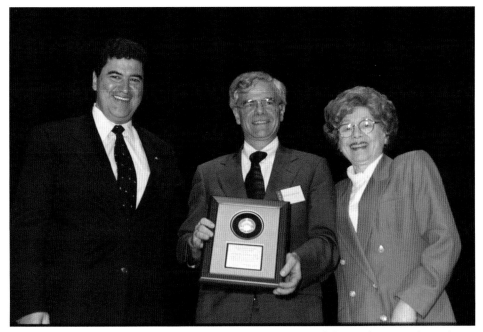

At the NIH Director's Awards Ceremony in June 2002, NIH principal deputy director Ruth Kirschstein and I stood with awardee and deputy director for intramural research Michael Gottesman. *Public domain from the NIH*

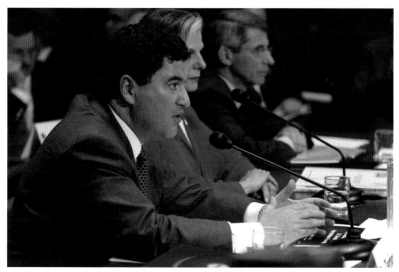

April 2003. As NIH director, I was testifying for the Senate Committee on Health, Education, Labor, and Pensions regarding the outbreak of severe acute respiratory syndrome. Beside me was Julie Gerberding, director of the U.S. Centers for Disease Control and Prevention, and Tony Fauci, director of the National Institute of Allergy and Infectious Diseases. *Getty Images/Douglas Graham/Contributor*

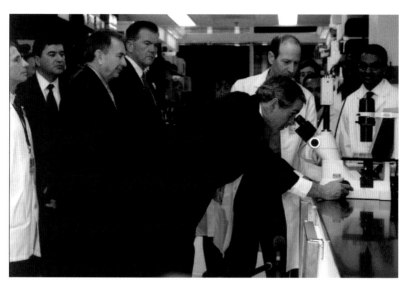

President Bush toured the Vaccine Research Center (VRC) in 2003, accompanied by (from left) NIAID director Tony Fauci, me, secretary of the Department of Health and Human Services Tommy Thompson, and secretary of the Department of Homeland Security Tom Ridge. Standing directly next to the president was VRC director Gary Nabel. *Public domain from the NIH (https://www.nih.gov/about-nih/what-we -do/nih-almanac/photo-gallery)*

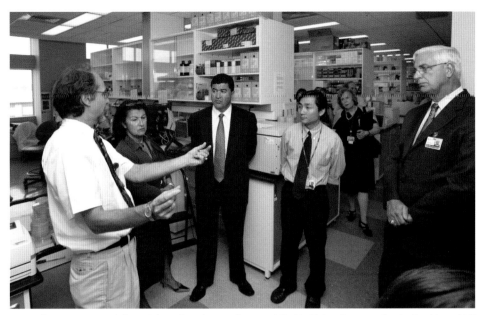

December 2004. From left to right: Jef Boeke, Nadia, me, Min Li, Elaine Freeman (in the back), and Ed Miller. The event was the opening of the High-Throughput Biology Center (of which Jef was a founding director), a pivotal interdisciplinary research center of the Johns Hopkins School of Medicine's Institute for Basic Biomedical Sciences. *Johns Hopkins University*

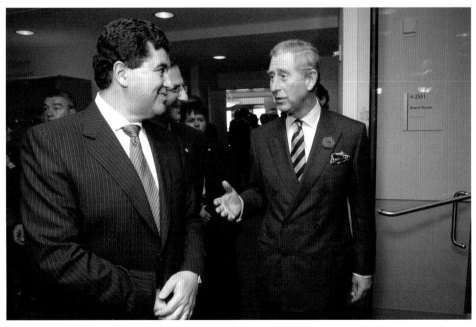

Here, I conversed with Prince Charles during a royal visit to the NIH in 2005. *Public domain from the NIH*

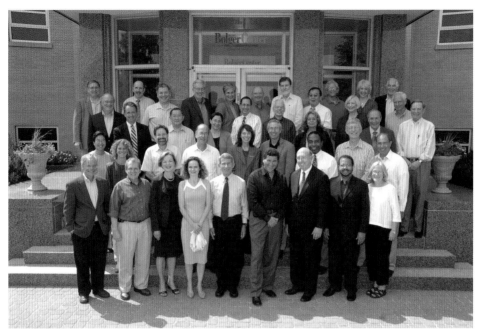

As NIH director, I joined institute and center directors and senior staff for a group photo in front of the Bolger Center in Potomac, Maryland, where we had gathered for a leadership forum. *Public domain from the NIH*

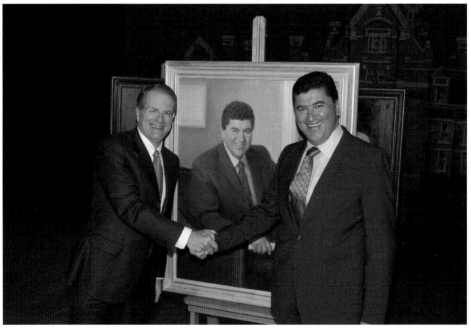

In 2007, Bill Brody, president of Johns Hopkins University, and me during my portrait dedication event at the university. *Robert J. Smith Jr.*

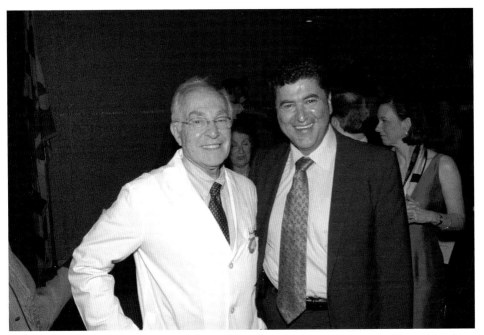

During my 2007 portrait dedication event at Johns Hopkins University, I stood for a photo with my long-time mentor and Hopkins radiology colleague, the brilliant Stan Siegelman. *Robert J. Smith Jr.*

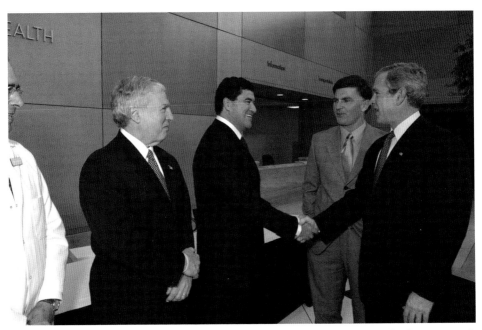

President Bush during a visit to the National Cancer Institute (NCI) in 2007. Maryland governor Bob Ehrlich was between the president and me. NCI director Andrew von Eschenbach was standing on my right. *Public domain from the NIH*

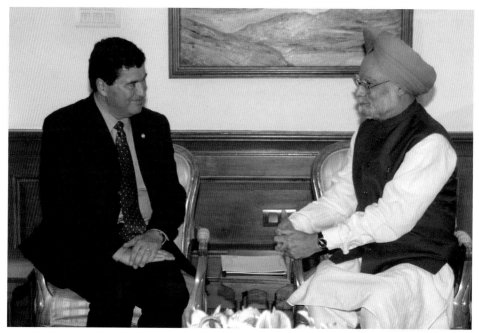

As NIH director, I was sitting down with Indian prime minister Manmohan Singh as part of a visit where we discussed HIV and other infectious disease research in India and in global health. *Public domain from the NIH*

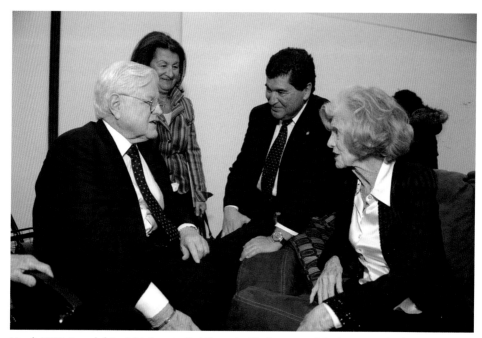

March 2008. From left to right: Senator Ted Kennedy, Nadia, me, and Eunice Kennedy Shriver. We were gathered to honor Shriver, whose monumental efforts had helped create the National Institute of Child Health and Human Development. In light of Eunice Kennedy Shriver's noble, tireless contributions, the institute had been newly renamed in her honor. *Public domain from the NIH*

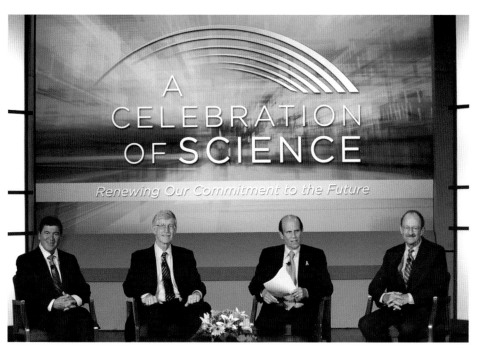

On Saturday, September 8, 2012, the NIH hosted a day of compelling presentations and "live remotes" as part of a three-day "Celebration of Science," in collaboration with FasterCures, the Milken Institute's Center for Accelerating Medical Solutions. Seated from left to right: me, NIH director Francis Collins, philanthropist and businessman Michael Milken, and former NIH director Harold Varmus. *NIH, https:// www.nih.gov/about-nih/who-we-are/nih-director/articles/celebration-science-nih, public domain from the NIH/FasterCures*

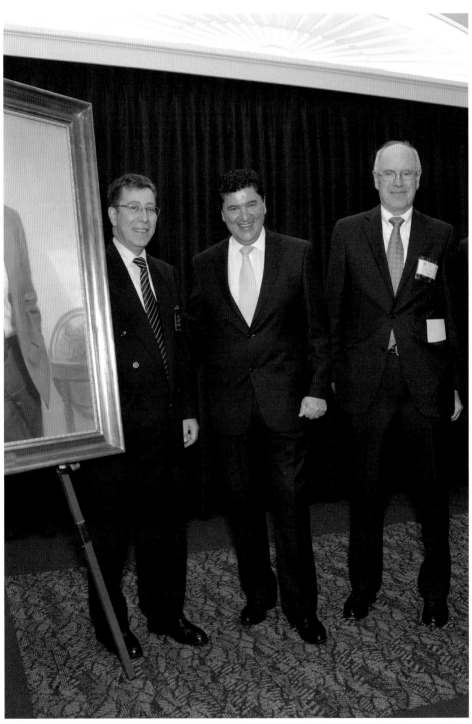

My brother Moustafa, Bruce Holbrook, and I were at the ceremony for the presentation of my portrait at the NIH in 2011. *Public domain from the NIH*

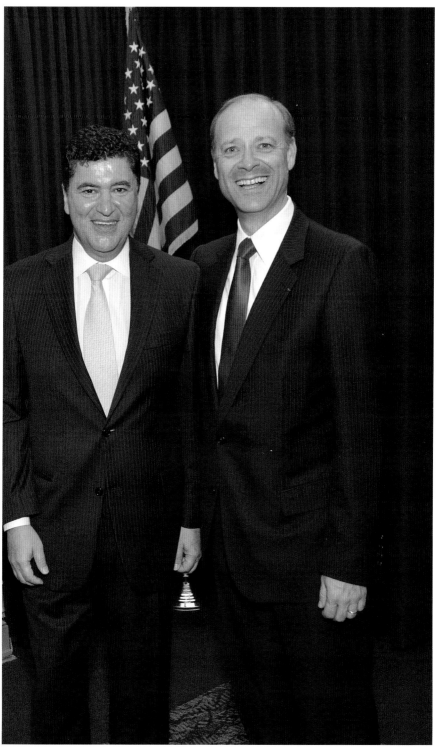

In 2011, Sanofi CEO Chris Viehbacher and I were at the ceremony for the presentation of my portrait at the NIH. *Public domain from the NIH*

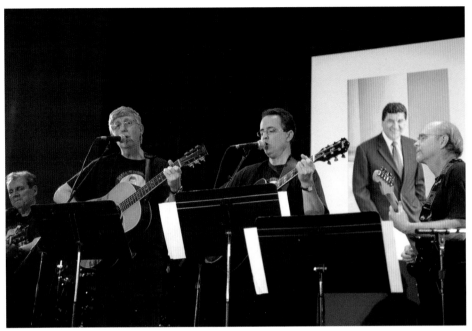

In 2008, during my farewell event at the NIH, I was treated to a performance by an excellent guitar band. From left to right: National Institute of Arthritis and Musculoskeletal and Skin Diseases (NIAMS) director Dr. Steve Katz, National Human Genome Research Institute director Francis Collins, NIH communications director John Burklow, and NIAMS scientific director John O'Shea. *Public domain from the NIH*

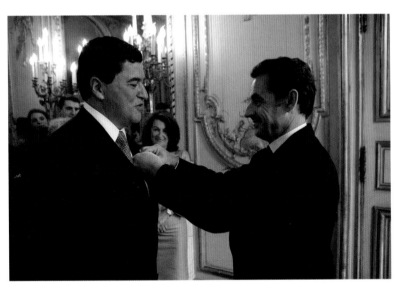

In 2008, in Paris, at the Élysée Palace, French president Nicolas Sarkozy pinned the Legion of Honour medal to my suit jacket as friends and family, including my wife, Nadia, and son, Will, looked on. *Arnaud Roiné/Présidence de la République*

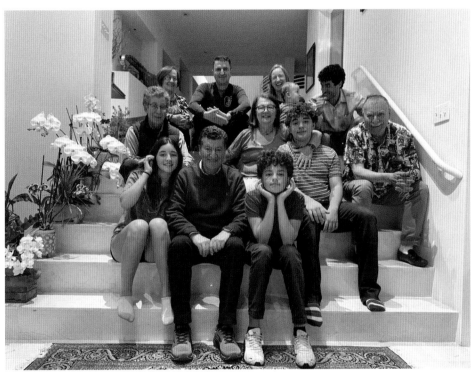

Taken in 2024 on my seventy-third birthday. I was happily surrounded by several generations of my family, including grandchildren. *Zerhouni family*

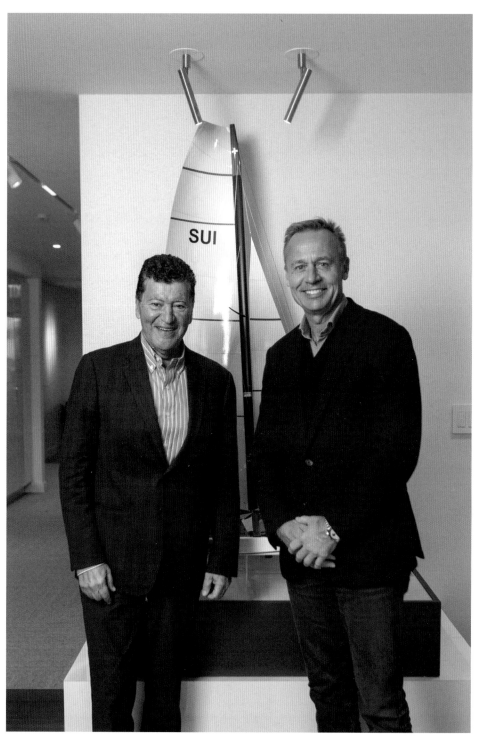

In October 2024, I visited Ernesto Bertarelli (cochair of the Bertarelli Foundation and chair of B-FLEXION) at his office in Boston, Massachusetts. *Kerry Goodwin*

whatever change is envisioned. Here again, integrity is a key ingredient to leadership.

～

On the day of the hearing, Senators Kennedy and Gregg arrived, and I introduced them to Nadia, my children, my now 83-year-old mother, and my longtime best friend from Algeria, Hachemi. It seemed like worlds ago that Hachemi and I had bonded in the classrooms of Lycee Emir Abdelkader in the years that followed the end of the war. Now here we were shaking hands with Senator Kennedy.

The hearing began. Ted Kennedy opened the proceedings. The senators of Maryland, Sarbanes and Mikulski, were seated by my side, ready to present me and support my nomination.

Senator Mikulski briefly went over my career. She described me as well fit to lead the NIH, as did Senator Sarbanes, who spoke next in support of me.

Senator Kennedy followed Sarbanes's remarks. He mentioned that my mother was in the audience and asked her to stand so that she could be welcomed and recognized. She was met with applause.

"We all know how important mothers are," Kennedy said.[1]

In his coming statements, Kennedy clearly established the stakes of the job of NIH director. The agency affected the lives of all Americans.

Kennedy explained, "NIH research ranges from studies of microscopic structures in living cells, to investigations of patterns of disease in entire populations. NIH research not only gives us information about what keeps us healthy or makes us sick, but it reveals new insights into who we are as human beings."[2]

Kennedy also mentioned great challenges the NIH faced. From developing new medicines to fight bioterrorism to helping restore confidence in clinical trials, the new NIH director would have their hands full.[3]

Kennedy's support for my nomination was evident. Regardless, I knew that I needed to properly deliver what would be my first testimony to Congress. As the hearing progressed and I drew closer to giving it, Republican senator John Warner spoke next.

"You're exhibit A regarding America's immigration policies. And it comes at a time when we are looking at those policies."[4]

Although this hearing may have been about the NIH, Warner's words highlighted the importance of the United States remaining open to immigration. If we close our doors, who might we be shutting out?

In my testimony, I shared my perspectives about what research should be in the coming century.[5] We needed to make new discoveries to facilitate the way we delivered health care, and we needed to more rapidly bring the fruits of our research to clinical testing.[6] I believed that biomedical research was at a turning point that might require new strategies, and to help illustrate this latter point, I used a novel DNA chip as a prop.[7]

"Amazingly, with one experiment, a scientist using this device can identify which of the thousands of human genes are active in any one biological sample," I explained. "Only a few years ago, it would have been impossible to ask the questions that we are able to explore with these revolutionary technologies."[8]

This DNA chip illustrated how technologies and knowledge from the physical and computational sciences were merging with molecular biology to enable deeper and larger-scale exploration of biological systems in health and disease.[9] It was just the beginning of an acceleration in fundamental research to understand the mechanisms of complex biological systems.[10] The second half of the twentieth century had witnessed an explosion of discoveries regarding the components of biological systems, such as DNA and RNA, yet we had made too little progress in our understanding of how all these numerous components interacted together to create life.[11]

As my next prop, I used a hypodermic needle.[12] Through it, I wanted to help demonstrate how much more progress we still needed to make and the immense scientific challenges of the day, including the enormous and poorly understood complexity of the microscopic world.[13]

"The tip of this needle is actually several times larger than any one single cell in the human body. Yet that single cell contains all of the human DNA, not just a subset, as in this DNA chip."[14]

That single cell also contained the entire molecular machinery necessary to transcribe and translate its DNA into all the complex networks of interacting molecules that make us what we are.[15]

We'd discovered most of the parts of our biological systems, and now we needed to go on a journey to understand how all these parts fit together in health and in disease.[16] This was by far the most formidable scientific problem ever faced by mankind.[17]

Scientific progress would increasingly depend on multidisciplinary teams.[18] When it came to the scientists themselves, the NIH needed to continue to train, recruit, and retain the best talent in biomedical research.[19] It was the creative spark of the unique individual that led to new knowledge and real progress.[20]

As my testimony continued, I brought up how new scientific knowledge could have the potential to raise deep moral issues.[21] Throughout history, tensions had always developed between science and society whenever a discovery challenged deeply held beliefs, and the resulting debates were polarizing.[22] What role then would I, as NIH director, play when such debates arose?[23]

"First and foremost, I believe that disease knows no politics. The NIH is a public agency at the vanguard of the fight against disease and is to serve all of us. I believe that the NIH director should not be or made to be, factional, but must always remain factual."[24]

I went on to address key issues such as stem cell research head-on rather than waiting for questions that could be formulated in leading ways.[25] Regarding President Bush's stem cell research policy, I underscored that it was an important advance: for the first time, NIH funding was allowed for such research.[26]

I expressed that, as director, I needed to reestablish morale, momentum, and a vision within the NIH as well as an energy to recruit exceptional individuals to key open positions.[27] I also needed to try to work with Congress and all other key parties to better understand the dynamics of research and research resources.[28] We needed to try to match the research resources we were given with the capacities of the system, the opportunities in science, the most creative scientists and engineers, and the priorities that were simultaneously set.[29]

In terms of changes I wanted to see, given the evolution of science, I felt it was important for the new NIH director to enhance crosscutting initiatives.[30] The director also needed to identify what the bottlenecks were for science today.[31] What was thwarting it?[32] For example, we needed to allow scientists throughout the country to have access to national resources that would facilitate their research.[33] Additionally, this research needed to be translated into a clinical reality.[34]

One of Kennedy's questions, which mentioned the newly created NIBIB, prompted me to assert that the NIH was facing a profound issue: the agency had difficulties promoting and developing areas of science that were crosscutting between institutes.[35] Although I didn't state it at this moment, I felt that the NIH needed to move from a structure of institutes specific to organs, groups of diseases, and so on to a much more open, crosscutting approach, inclusive of emerging technologies.[36] Breaking the historical barriers between the fields of science and their entrenched disciplines would be a priority for me.[37]

I recognized that achieving this change in a successful agency like the NIH would be difficult.[38] Forming a system of support designed to be more inclusive of non-biomedical disciplines would require a cultural shift.[39] I was comfortable with that prospect, having experienced the benefits of an open, multidisciplinary approach with my research at Hopkins.[40] However, would NIH scientists be open to a realignment of scientific priorities if it meant that budgets would no longer be wholly directed to their interests?[41]

The hearing shifted as Senator Wellstone asked questions.[42] With his words, Wellstone again showed his deep commitment to the cause of battling muscular dystrophy.[43] Eventually, he brought up stem cell research, pressing me on the subject.[44]

"If necessary, will you recommend that the President's [stem cell] policy be broadened to include additional lines?" Wellstone asked.[45]

To this question, I responded, "[If] it becomes evident through this research that there are pathways to develop cures . . . I will be the first one to assemble that information, to get the experts to give that information, to provide that in the sense of well-established scientific facts and share that with everyone."[46]

In my answer, I was walking a political tightrope while speaking true to what I would do as director. Wellstone wasn't satisfied.[47]

"I appreciate it [your answer]," he said. "I am not sure whether it was a 'yes' or 'no' answer, and I am not a scientist, so I appreciate it—I am in politics and public affairs—but I do not think it was quite the commitment that I was hoping to hear, but I will follow up with you on it; okay?"[48]

"That would be fine."[49]

Wellstone was a modest, noble public servant who fought for vulnerable Americans. Tragically, he would die in a plane crash in October 2002. He would be missed.

After Wellstone finished speaking and some further questioning was completed, Senator Kennedy closed the hearing.[50]

"Our country is very fortunate, and the nation is, the world is, to have his [Dr. Zerhouni's] services to lead this great institution."[51]

I was confirmed by a unanimous consent vote on May 2, 2002, becoming the fifteenth director of the NIH.

Building a Roadmap for Twenty-First-Century Medical Research 16

In July 2003, the *New York Times* would publish an interview with me. "What does it take to be a leader?" I was asked.[1]

> I think there are three things. First you have to have a big heart. Because if you don't have a big heart you will never be able to lead. And a big heart means several things to me. You have to have a passion. You have to believe in some things that are your core values. The second is you have to have a spine, which means stand up for what you think and take the risks that you think are important. And third and least important is brains. People often think that high intelligence is a prerequisite. I don't believe so. I think a big heart and a strong spine are more important than high intelligence.[2]

~

After being confirmed as NIH director, I knew I'd need heart, spine, and brain to succeed. At Hopkins, I'd had four jobs at once. Now I would have one job that was more complicated than having five at once.

As part of my transition into the directorship, I had to find a way to leave Hopkins in good standing despite having little time to do so. To complicate matters, after being confirmed, there were plenty of requests for briefings to bring me up to speed on what was going on at the NIH. Some briefings were focused on key, controversial issues, including embryonic stem cell research.

Accepting the directorship also forced me to divest any shares in companies that could create a conflict of interest. It was a large but necessary sacrifice that allowed me to be unbiased and free of industry influence.

Despite obstacles, I navigated my transition into government, officially starting my tenure on May 20, 2002. In my new office, I was sworn in. There was no large ceremony.

I immediately began my work, adjusting to my new office commute and the extensive, post-9/11 security. Meanwhile, some in the scientific community questioned whether I should have been appointed director in the first place. Their reasons were grounded in prejudice. They believed that because I was a radiologist, I didn't know enough about basic science. To quote Bill Brody, this was like saying that because Bill Gates was a programmer, he didn't know anything about business.[3]

My critics were wrong. I had the knowledge and experience needed to succeed. Even still, it wouldn't be easy. I'd inherited an agency facing serious challenges. There was much to be done, and as a leader, I knew that being proactive was always key.

~

The month of May was a relatively quiet time at the NIH, as the budget had already been approved. I reviewed it and sat down with Ruth Kirschstein, who'd been the acting NIH director. In a remarkable career in public service, Ruth had loyally and passionately served the NIH in different capacities for decades. Her integrity and dedication to the agency was an inspiration, as was her commitment to scientists from minority backgrounds.

Ruth and I met regularly to discuss agency issues. We enjoyed a productive relationship. Her advice was invaluable. She showed me the skeletons in the closet and told me where the land mines were hidden.

I'd inherited an NIH facing serious problems. There was much to be done. The clock was ticking. Being proactive was key. Yet the NIH didn't have a clear path forward.

I met with the directors of the institutes to help identify who the key opinion leaders were. At our first large meeting, I introduced myself. They didn't know me personally. I learned later that the institute directors and their staff had been calling me "Zer Who?"

I identified the key leaders that everyone followed. Francis Collins, director of the National Human Genome Research Institute (NHGRI), was one of them. A man of science and God, he would one day go on to become an excellent NIH director. Tony Fauci, director of NIAID, was another leader within the NIH. I would come to admire Fauci's ability to put the interests of the NIH above his own. He was always willing to sacrifice for the greater good of the institution.

I would work closely with him for seven years. He always served public health through the best science, whether in combating AIDS, tuberculosis, malaria, Ebola, flu, or COVID-19. Without the research he supported in his institute over the years, we would not have been able to develop a vaccine against COVID-19 in nine months, an unprecedented achievement in the history of medicine. I consider him one of the best civil servants and scientists this country has ever had.

Regarding exceptional civil servants, Thomas Insel, who would head the National Institute of Mental Health from the fall of 2002 until 2015, was another leader at the NIH whom I would come to respect greatly. Well beyond the end of his tenure, Thomas would carry on his tireless, impactful battle for bettering the mental health of all Americans.

~

During my early days as director, I received a visit from a White House lawyer.

"Be careful on the stem cell issue. You need to support the president's policy."

The lawyer had been hearing noise that I might diverge from it. I reassured him I wouldn't.

"I'll report objectively on the science. The president is the one making the policy decisions."

> Seemingly satisfied, the lawyer then told me, "I've seen a lot of agency directors. They keep busy with details. And then time flies. And at the end of their tenure, they look back and say, 'What have I accomplished?,' and they realize it's nothing. . . . I advise you to think in two- or three-year terms at most. You don't know if the President will be reelected. So, whatever you want to do, get it done now."

Time was of the essence. I knew that I needed to bring the institutes together for the purpose of accomplishing that which none of them could on their own. However, I didn't yet know what the institutes needed to collectively focus on. The road forward wasn't mapped out. Meanwhile, as I would explain in an article I wrote for *Science*, the agency's budget increase (reaching more than $27 billion by 2003) would speed up the pace of scientific discovery and heighten public expectations.[4] The NIH needed to deliver.

I spoke to our director of policy, Lana Skirboll, an astute and hard-working neuroscientist. I wanted her team to develop a strategic plan for medical research. John Burklow, my invaluable associate director for communications, was also present.

"Please don't use the word strategic plan," Lana insisted.

"Why?" I asked.

"Because one of the past NIH directors tried to do a strategic plan, and it was a disaster."

"Okay. Let's call it the roadmap, instead."

It would be known as the NIH Roadmap for Medical Research, and, as I explained to the scientific community in my October 2003 article for *Science*, "The NIH Roadmap," it would be focused on efforts that no single or small group of institutes or centers could or should conduct on its own.[5] As I stated in my article, science was converging on a set of unifying principles that linked seemingly disparate diseases through common biological pathways and therapeutic approaches, and NIH research needed to reflect this new reality.[6]

We needed actionable, feasible goals and priorities. Before deciding what priorities would be addressed in the roadmap, I wanted to have a series of meetings with key opinion leaders from both the institutes and outside the NIH. Their input would be fundamental in shaping what we assembled.

Meanwhile, our warp-speed work tempo would ensure that the roadmap was assembled sooner rather than later. When I told Lana Skirboll and John Burklow that we had to have it assembled by September 1, 2002, they looked at me like I was crazy.

"It can be done," I assured them. "I'll show you how. I'll work with you."

I would earn the nickname "Warp Speed Director," replacing my former one, "Zer Who?"

As I would later explain in my 2003 article for *Science*, to help assemble the roadmap, we invited more than 300 of the nation's biomedical leaders, from academia, government, and the private sector, to Washington, spread across several meetings, throughout the course of the summer of 2002.[7] We asked participants to address three key questions: (1) What are today's most pressing scientific challenges? (2) What are the roadblocks to progress, and what must be done to overcome them? (3) Which efforts are beyond the mandate of one or a few institutes but the responsibility of NIH as a whole?[8]

Some of my staff felt we wouldn't be able to get many of the leaders we invited to come to Washington in the middle of the summer. To my surprise, almost all of them agreed to come. Only one turned us down due to a family vacation. The high participation rate was a good sign. There was a hunger for clarity and purpose from the NIH.

The meetings were successful, and the number of recommendations for the roadmap was enormous. We had around 900. We couldn't pursue them all. We needed to identify which were most important.

"Look, let me tell you my philosophy when it comes to this," I told my staff. "It's called Rock, Pebble, Sand."

They looked at me like I was out of this world. What was Rock, Pebble, Sand?

Imagine I put an empty vase on a table next to a pile of rocks, a pile of pebbles, and a pile of sand. In what order would you put these contents into the empty vase so that they fit inside it as compactly as possible? What would be your strategy? You'll realize that the best way is to put in the rocks first, followed by the pebbles, and then the sand. Rock, Pebble, Sand is a metaphor for prioritization.

It's also a way by which you can identify and understand the real drivers of possible change in any system. What are the rocks that would create the most positive change? Move them into the jar first.

I didn't come up with the Rock, Pebble, Sand metaphor. Yet I love using it.

Having explained the metaphor to my staff, I told them to go back and classify every roadmap recommendation into a rock category, pebble category, or sand category. I wanted them to identify what recommendations were most fundamental. The institute directors, whom I'd appointed to chair the meetings so they could participate in listening to their constituencies, worked with my staff to determine which category recommendations fell under.

We ended up with 98 rocks. This number was still too high. The NIH couldn't pursue them all.

At an agency retreat with the institute directors present, I had them assess which rocks were high priority. We organized a voting mechanism. It helped in eliminating some rocks, yet we still had too many.

During an evening at the retreat, I thought of a different strategy. I classified what I saw as the fundamental issues among the rocks. I categorized the rocks into families. The next day of the retreat, I met with my colleagues.

"I see a pattern. Among the rocks, three themes emerge."

They were (1) New Pathways to Discovery, (2) Reengineering the Clinical Research Enterprise, and (3) Research Teams of the Future.[9] The foundation of the roadmap had been identified.

~

The Rock, Pebble, Sand metaphor helped us arrive at this conclusion, and it wouldn't be the last time I used it as director. It would be a regular part of my process. For example, at staff meetings, I'd ask employees to classify a certain issue as a rock, a pebble, or sand.

At times, I'd classify an issue myself and ask if they agreed with my thinking. Incorporating this philosophy was a powerful way of motivating the team to focus on key priorities. It also helped me avoid unnecessary micromanagement, as I identified "sand" issues that arrived in meetings and delegated the responsibility of taking care of them. This gave me more time to focus on priority issues.

~

After developing the NIH Roadmap for Medical Research, I had to obtain the funding for the initiatives. A strategy without a budget is nothing, just as a budget without a strategy is nothing.

As I stated in my 2003 article for *Science*, the roadmap's three themes were examined by 15 working groups, led by institute directors, with input from the NIH Council of Public Representatives and the Advisory Committee to the Director.[10] Meanwhile, as we moved forward with building the roadmap, discovery in the life sciences continued to accelerate at an unprecedented rate, and the recently completed sequencing of the human genome (thanks in part to the leadership of NHGRI director Francis Collins) presented both opportunities and challenges, the latter of which would redefine the ways that medical research would be conducted and lead to improvements in health.[11]

In June 2003, NIH leadership convened to select roadmap initiatives to launch in 2004, basing decisions off key criteria questions, such as, is the initiative truly transforming—will it dramatically change the content or the process of medical research in the next decade?[12]

Our 15 working groups evolved into nine implementation groups tasked with developing their proposals into tangible activities.[13] Collaboration remained key.

~

The roadmap's program plans were well received by Congress. However, within the larger scientific community, the response was mixed. It seemed like roughly 60 percent of scientists were neutral. Of the remaining 40 percent, half were negative, and half were positive.

As I was working with Congress and further assembling the plans, more opposition from the scientific community emerged. I responded by holding my ground. I told them I was not going to change my mind because what they were objecting to was not my idea. It was built from the ideas of their own community. The roadmap had been born from consensus rather than from the will of one person.

I'd long believed that the way to tackle opposition was to bring in data and transparency. As illustrated in chapter 13, it had proved useful when dealing with the issue of research space at Hopkins. If one brought in data and transparency in a way that was not confrontational, not "my way or the highway," they often prevailed.

When it came to the roadmap, we were able to change the minds of some of our opponents. Yet there were those who remained completely and viciously opposed. They leveled personal attacks at me. Even still, I held my ground.

I learned a key rule of leadership through this experience. If you seek significant reform, no matter what it is, you'll always face opposition from those who feel they stand to lose. You're changing the status quo and disturbing special interests.

It's essential to properly manage the inevitable conflict that comes from pursuing and enacting reform. Understand that many individuals will not sacrifice for the greater good without some sort of compensation or a chance to sustain themselves. It's not their fault. They are acting in accordance with human nature.

To complicate matters, the gains that individuals stand to make from reforms might manifest only in the long term, while the sacrifices can be immediate. How does a leader convince others to embrace a reform if it will hurt them today and help them years from now? This is a question every leader must ask themselves.

During the roadmap experience, I also learned that it isn't wise to waffle or change your plans because of opposition. If you do, you're telling the opposition they are right, emboldening them further. Your supporters become less supportive, and your adversaries become more powerful. If you are not willing to stand up firmly for what you propose to do, why would anybody follow you?

~

One of the issues we faced in putting together the roadmap was finding the money for its initiatives. Ultimately, it was funded through "voluntary" (meaning firmly requested) contributions from the NIH's institutes and centers and supplemented by direct appropriations from the Office of the Director.[14] At the beginning of the roadmap, we had a small budget to fund the common purposes of the agency. As this common fund grew over time, it would transform the way the agency functioned for joint projects that the NIH needed to carry out but that no single institute could or would.

Some prominent scientists and advocates immediately understood the importance of supporting the roadmap. One of them was the hardworking and transformative philanthropist Michael Milken, who asked to visit me. I did not know him personally, though I knew of him. He was a controversial financial genius who had become a tireless and creative advocate for cancer research.

When Michael came to my office, he wanted to know how to best help the NIH forward (and to assess me, I surmised). He had carefully studied the issues facing prostate cancer research, as he had been diagnosed with it. He thought in terms of Rock, Pebble, and Sand, just like I did. As we talked, I observed that he was visionary in his approach to changes that the system needed. I was intrigued by his way of analyzing issues.

Over the years, Michael would remain a staunch and effective advocate for the NIH and biomedical research. Following my NIH tenure, we would become good friends. I would be particularly touched by his dedication to preserving the American dream. Michael was a man who'd remade his life in the service of others.

~

When it came to serving the nation, regarding the roadmap, I informed Congress that we wanted them to see the current iteration of the common fund as a pilot experiment for how the NIH could be better run. Senator Kennedy was supportive. Senator Judd Gregg was as well.

Through the NIH Roadmap's umbrella of initiatives (New Pathways to Discovery, Reengineering the Clinical Research Enterprise, and Research Teams of the Future) came a variety of meaningful programs.[15]

Within New Pathways to Discovery, initiatives addressed the technologies and approaches necessary to meet research challenges, including molecular imaging, the development of small-molecule libraries, bioinformatics and computational biology, nanomedicine, and structural biology.[16] When it came to Reengineering the Clinical Research Enterprise, an immense challenge, the NIH would promote the creation of better-integrated networks of academic centers that would work jointly on clinical trials and include community-based physicians.[17] The NIH would design pilot programs for a revolutionary National Electronic Clinical Trials and Research network, which would begin to develop an informatics infrastructure that would link current and emerging clinical research information systems so that data and resources could be shared within and across clinical research networks, across studies, and across institutions, reducing duplication and avoiding unnecessary overlap between trials.[18] Regarding Research Teams of the Future, we aimed to accelerate movement of scientific discoveries from the bench to the patient's bedside, encouraging novel public and private partnerships as well as nontraditional multidisciplinary scientist teams and high-risk, high-reward research.[19] Additionally, young scientists would benefit from the roadmap, as it would encourage their exploration and growth.

Yet no one would benefit more than the American people. In assembling this roadmap, we made sure their needs were paramount. All Americans, regardless of race, creed, and politics, were our constituency. Their public health problems were ours to face.

One of the most significant developments in the NIH's history, the roadmap was a six-year, $2.2 billion blueprint that the institutes and centers responded to with amazing speed, as more than a year after the roadmap's official launch (September 30, 2003), it was right on schedule.[20] Yet some remained skeptical as to whether the roadmap would endure beyond my tenure. Funding was built largely on voluntary contributions from the institutes and centers. To survive, the common fund needed to be drawn directly from the government. Additionally, for the fund to fulfill the vision of the roadmap, it needed to be far larger. There was still work to be done.

The Gates Foundation, Congress, and the U.S. President's Emergency Plan for AIDS Relief

17

Early in my tenure, former NCI director Rick Klausner visited me. He was now the executive director of the global health program at the Bill & Melinda Gates Foundation. He'd developed the idea of Grand Challenges in Global Health: significant "scientific challenges that, if solved, could lead to key advances in preventing, treating, and curing the diseases and health conditions contributing most to global health inequity."[1] The effort was conceptually similar to that of mathematician David Hilbert at the beginning of the twentieth century as he defined 23 Grand Challenges in mathematics, thus propelling the field forward.

Rick Klausner and Bill Gates felt the foundation needed to define what the Grand Challenges in Global Health were and then support the task of overcoming them. Unfortunately, the Gates Foundation lacked the infrastructure, staff, and experience needed to independently pull this off. Rick felt that teaming with the NIH could help solve these problems.

During his visit with me, Rick expressed a desire to have me work alongside the Gates Foundation in defining the Grand Challenges.

"I want a yes or no, not a maybe. Okay?" Rick said, echoing my request years prior, when he'd approached me to work with the NCI.

I was happy to help with the Grand Challenges, yet I needed to see if I could. Soon, NIH's general counsel informed me that I couldn't work with a private foundation. I was frustrated. Yet I wasn't giving up.

There was a nonprofit organization called the Foundation for the NIH (FNIH) that could be helpful. The foundation was created by Congress in 1990 to organize and direct public–private collaborations and alliances that promoted transformative scientific research and enhanced quality of life. I believed it was possible to have the FNIH help with the

Grand Challenges without violating any laws. Wanting to move forward, I contacted Rick Klausner.

"How much money are you willing to put into this?" I asked.

"$200 million."

After discussing the opportunity with the FNIH's chair, Charles Sanders, and the FNIH's executive director and CEO, Amy McGuire Porter, both of whom were supportive, I told Rick the foundation would work with him. Yet since the FNIH didn't have much money, the Gates Foundation would have to foot the bill.

"So, how much do you want for FNIH to do it?" Rick asked.

Institutions usually charged 15 or 20 percent to do the work of a grant. We ultimately agreed on 11 percent. The head of the FNIH was overjoyed. With that money, the foundation could be built up. Together, the FNIH and the Gates Foundation moved forward.

In seeking to identify the Grand Challenges, we sourced ideas from the scientific community while utilizing a stellar international (incorporating some developing countries) selection panel comprised of 20 scientists and public health experts.[2] Our selection panel had an executive committee that included Harold Varmus, Rick, and myself. Harold was our chair, while Rick and I cochaired.

Our panel hashed out what the Grand Challenges in Global Health were. We ended up with 14, connected to seven general objectives: improving childhood vaccines, creating new vaccines, controlling insects that transmit agents of disease, improving nutrition to promote health, improving drug treatment of infectious diseases, curing latent and chronic infections, and measuring disease and health status accurately and economically in developing countries.[3] In an October 2003 article in *Science* that I coauthored with Harold, Rick, Tara Acharya, Abdallah Daar, and Peter Singer, we thoughtfully outlined these goals, providing a detailed account of how we arrived at them and how we aimed to move forward, issuing "Request for Proposals (RFP) to address each of the challenges with grants of up to a total of $20 million over 5 years or less."[4]

This initial Grand Challenges initiative eventually awarded $450 million worth of grants.[5] Bill Gates's dedicated, transformative philanthropy was inspiring. The Gates funding helped put the FNIH on the map as an effective integrator of public and private initiatives, setting it on a path to great success in bringing additional resources to support the NIH mission.

Despite initial worries from NIH general council, the Grand Challenges program had been a success story for the FNIH. I was glad it had moved forward.

In facing difficult decisions, since my medical school days in Algeria, I'd always asked myself, what is the worst that could happen? As I said in chapter 5, for making decisions that involve a degree of risk, using the worst-case scenario as a basis for whether one should proceed is prudent. If one can live with the worst outcome, then why not proceed?

In the case of taking on the Grand Challenges through the FNIH, President Bush wouldn't fire me for encouraging a program that was so valuable and good in its intentions. I also wouldn't be sued by anyone, as I wasn't taking any actions that were illegal. So why not move forward?

~

As director, I moved forward with building relationships with key decision-makers in Congress.

"You need to get to know the relevant members of Congress and spend time with them and their staff," Marc Smolonsky, my legislative aide, advised. "And the best way is to visit their own state or district while they are in the minority, not when they're in the majority. You need to visit the guys in the majority for sure. But visit the other ones too."

Following Marc's advice, I spent time meeting with legislators on both sides of the aisle. I didn't come to them with a problem that needed their attention. Instead, I visited when I didn't need anything from them. I got to know them, and they got to know me, without agendas.

I visited them in their home districts. This was where they preferred to be visited. Having the NIH director come to announce a grant to their local university was a big plus for them.

One of the senators I spent time with was Ted Kennedy. Our relationship had started off on a strong note during my confirmation process. Over time, we became good friends.

"Would you come with me to the University of Massachusetts [UMass]?" the senator asked me one day. "We just gave them a grant, and I want to show support."

Together, the senator and I went to Baltimore/Washington International Airport. As part of the heightened, post-9/11 security, at the gate, they would pick certain passengers for a second security check. It was supposedly random. As Senator Kennedy and I arrived at the gate, the security agent pointed his finger at one of us, signaling for that person to come over to him. Being an Arab American, I assumed it was me. I approached the security agent while Kennedy stayed behind, assuming the same thing I had.

"No, no, no. Not you," the agent told me. "You, sir." He pointed to Senator Kennedy.

We were surprised. They were going to do a second security check on Ted Kennedy?

Afterward, the senator and I laughed.

"Senator, I thought it was for me."

"Yeah. I thought it was for you, too."

Eventually, Senator Kennedy and I arrived at UMass. The institution had done an excellent job of growing its basic research. An example of this progress was the recent work of the brilliant Dr. Craig Mello. One of the reasons I'd visited UMass was to receive a briefing from Dr. Mello about his co-discovery of a process called RNA interference. The breakthrough would soon earn him and Andrew Fire a well-deserved Nobel Prize. Kennedy and I were briefed on the discovery, taking in Dr. Mello's words with great interest.

Later, as Kennedy and I continued our visit, I sought to better understand the effect of the NIH on state institutions like UMass. How had UMass, which hadn't been known for basic science, made such a leap? Two key drivers behind this leap were the great, visionary leadership of the university president, William Bulger, and the budget increase that came from the NIH.

After the visit, Senator Kennedy and I drove back to Boston together. During the trip, Kennedy told me that the brother of the president of UMass was an infamous gangster named Whitey Bulger. The senator and I laughed at the absurdity of this, and we bonded during our car ride.

I brought up the issue of the growing partisanship I was observing in Congress. Kennedy agreed that relationships had changed and were less congenial across the aisle than they had been. He bemoaned the rise of gerrymandering, detrimental to our democracy. He pointed out, however, that somehow the country had always found a way forward in times of challenge, citing civil rights and voting rights legislation of the 1950s and 1960s.

"Never doubt the ability of America to do the right thing eventually," Kennedy said.

He proceeded to drive me to see my son, Will, at Harvard Law School.

The close relationship Kennedy and I forged would prove pivotal later in my tenure during the challenges of the NIH Reform Act of 2006.

Kennedy would often call me at home to discuss NIH matters. Nadia would pick up.

"Naaadia!" he'd kindly say with his Massachusetts accent.

∽

While the NIH directorship kept me busy, Nadia adjusted with difficulty to having a spouse working in a demanding, high-level government role that included serious media scrutiny and challenging constraints. Since I was no longer in academia, Nadia and I were now swimming in different streams. At Hopkins, we'd been part of a big family. Now Nadia wasn't included.

I traveled regularly and at times was overwhelmed with tasks. As a result, I saw Nadia and my children far less than I wanted to. When I did see them, the Blackberry phone I carried with me would constantly alert me of some task or problem that needed my attention.

Nadia continued to be an extraordinary mother to our children while also propelling her own career forward. She was still working in pediatric endocrinology at Hopkins while also helping with international adoption services.

∽

Before I became NIH director, President Bush was looking to help HIV patients in Africa on the recommendation of Tony Fauci and several presidential advisers at the White House. The epidemic in Africa had reached frightening proportions. Across the continent, countless Africans were dying.

Medications for HIV were expensive and not accessible everywhere. Essentially, the rich world had them, and the poor world didn't. Nations with few resources, notably those in sub-Saharan Africa, were stricken with HIV infections, and antiretroviral medications were not readily available.[6] Another part of the problem was inadequate disease prevention.

Mike Gerson, a powerful adviser and speechwriter at the White House, and NIAID director Tony Fauci and other close advisers helped convince President Bush to act and include what would be a truly transformative initiative in the fight against HIV in his State of the Union Address.[7] Some prominent conservatives were against the move, as were the Office of Management and Budget representatives, yet President Bush, to his credit, refused to back down. As a born-again Christian, he believed helping Africa with its epidemic was the right thing to do. The U.S. President's Emergency Plan for AIDS Relief (PEPFAR) was envisioned.

∽

The PEPFAR program was announced on January 28, 2003. Bush ordered a team to visit Africa to assess PEPFAR's feasibility. The returning report was positive, and the Bush administration directed NIAID's Mark Dybul and Tony Fauci to design the PEPFAR program.[8] Delivering crucial medications to HIV-infected patients in Africa and the Caribbean and providing methods of disease prevention were key objectives of the program, which was authorized on May 27, 2003.[9]

In December 2003, Secretary Thompson led a special delegation, which included CDC director Julie Gerberding, Tony Fauci, and me, among others, to Africa. We aimed to examine the on-the-ground efforts of the newly established PEPFAR program and further needs in the battle against HIV. We also sought to put a spotlight on the epidemic, opening eyes to its horrors.[10] Accordingly, the delegation was a large collection of key professionals, including some from nongovernmental organizations, such as Pharma executives.

GlaxoSmithKline's Chris Viehbacher was someone I conversed with on the plane ride over. I got to know him. Chris would play a large role in my life years later after he became CEO of the multinational pharmaceutical giant Sanofi.

After arriving in Africa, we visited countries that were being hit the hardest by HIV. During the trip, I bonded with Secretary Thompson, who was gregarious and friendly. He was also unbelievably hardworking. Although in his early sixties, he had the energy of a young man. He seemed to work from seven in the morning until two at night and then start over again the next day. I admired his drive and work ethic.

The delegation arrived at a village in Kenya where Secretary Thompson was supposed to give a talk and present a gift. Regarding the latter, Thompson had inquired as to what was the most precious gift to give. It turned out that in these poor villages, it was a cow that gave milk. With this, one could feed their children.

Thompson was from Wisconsin. He arranged to have a cow transported from his home state to Kenya. It was presented as a gift to the village. I had tears in my eyes as I saw it unfold. It was such a thoughtful, generous act.

"This is a great man," I said to myself.

Our delegation traveled to villages in Uganda that had been hit hard by HIV. We saw poor farms, with grandparents taking care of numerous grandchildren. The parents were dead. I saw their tombs around the farms. It was heartbreaking.

The delegation's travels also included Cameroon, Zambia, Rwanda, and Tanzania. We saw that in much of Africa, there was inadequate infrastructure. People would have to walk 20 miles to reach a clinic. This made it hard to distribute medicine.

However, we discovered that locals had already found a solution in the form of Toyota motorcycles that could drive onto dirt roads. Toyota had donated many of these motorcycles, leading to their use for shuttling HIV medications along difficult dirt routes. With this mode of transportation, patients far from the cities could be reached. I saw this as a sign that PEPFAR could succeed with the right transportation mechanisms in place. After we returned from our trip to Africa, we gave our report to the president.

PEPFAR would, as the U.S. government stated, be the largest commitment by any nation to address a single disease in history. Following Mark Dybul's outstanding tenure leading the program, among other champions and stewards of PEPFAR, Dr. Deborah Birx and her efforts as the director of CDC's Division of Global HIV/AIDS and as U.S. global AIDS coordinator would be invaluable.

Decades later, with PEPFAR ongoing, it would be estimated that 25 million lives had been saved by the program.[11] PEPFAR earned America a great deal of goodwill in African countries. It's a lesson in the value of soft power and generosity versus hard power and violence. It's often better to influence the world by transforming health rather than blowing up buildings.

Bioterrorism, Pandemic Threats, and a Conflict-of-Interest Crisis

18

A week after 9/11, letters carrying anthrax spores started arriving at their intended destinations. The worst biological attacks in American history resulted in the deaths of five Americans and the illness of seventeen more.[1]

Bioterrorism was a public health emergency. Accordingly, some of the NIH budget was shifted toward it. NIAID and its director, Tony Fauci, took the lead on bioterrorism and helped launch project Bioshield (to be added to NIAID's budget and missions).

After committing substantial funds to bioterrorism research, in time, the NIH was asked to commit even more. The government wanted to stockpile an anthrax vaccine. Congress ordered the NIH to buy the stockpile for a colossal sum. If Congress kept ordering us to foot the bill for whatever bioterrorism-related purchase they needed to make, it could become a real problem for both the finances and the mission at the NIH.

Our mission wasn't to stockpile vaccines. In the case of bioterrorism, we ought to help in a research capacity. Tony Fauci and I discussed the issue and agreed that we needed to talk to Congress and maybe have another mechanism worked out. Maybe a separate agency could be created, we thought. Thanks to Tony's stature, excellent relationships with multiple presidential administrations, and experience, he was able to convince the current administration of the need to address this rising issue.

This is where having good relationships with senators such as Ted Kennedy and Judd Gregg and representatives such as Ralph Regula and Bill Young also helped. I went to see all of them in support of the idea of creating a separate agency for preparedness.

"I don't want to have NIH be a purchasing agent," I told Senator Gregg.

He agreed with me. Senator Gregg and others worked with Senator Richard Burr, who was also on the HELP Committee, to create a solution to our problem. Burr became the key legislative leader in introducing the Pandemic and All-Hazards Preparedness Act (PAHPA), which would become the law of the land at the end of 2006.[2] PAHPA's purpose would be "to improve the Nation's public health and medical preparedness and response capabilities for emergencies, whether deliberate, accidental, or natural."[3] As part of PAHPA, the Biomedical Advanced Research and Development Authority (BARDA) would be created at HHS, taking the burden of procurement away from the NIH. Meanwhile, the NIH would still be connected to bioterrorism in a research capacity, more in line with the fundamental mission of the agency.

∼

In 2003, severe acute respiratory syndrome (SARS), which originated in southern China (in 2002), caused a huge scare, spreading throughout the globe. In response, we worked closely with the CDC, the White House, and Congress. The breakout was controlled through effective public health techniques, including rapid diagnosis, patient isolations, epidemiological investigations, and quarantines of exposed persons.[4] Thankfully, the outbreak died off in six months. We learned our lesson from the experience. We needed a national plan to respond to pandemics. We set about making one.

In the conversations that shaped our pandemic plan, which involved key experts, I was a secondary player, as I wasn't as experienced in these issues as some of my colleagues, such as Tony Fauci.

To adequately combat pandemic threats and bioterrorism, the United States also needed strategic stockpile areas, accessible to transportation that could reach all Americans. We discovered that the United States Postal Service (USPS) was the best organization to fulfill the task of bringing countermeasures to all Americans. The USPS had the capacity to reach almost every American in a relatively short amount of time, making it a valuable tool in the event of a bioterrorism attack or pandemic.

The H5N1 flu was another pandemic scare we dealt with. The president discussed it during one of his visits to the NIH. We also talked about the national pandemic response plan, which, by then, we had nearly finished developing. President Bush and Vice President Dick Cheney had been involved in the process of putting it together.

The pandemic response plan we ended up with was excellent. The NIH was intrinsic to it, along with the CDC, then led by the accomplished, effective, and respected Dr. Julie Gerberding. I'd one day wish that the United States had kept the pandemic response plan in place and used it for COVID-19. Unfortunately, our plan would be put on a shelf and forgotten. There would be so many pandemic risks that came up as time went by —influenza, Ebola, and others. Repeated false alarms would create a fictional sense of security in the face of new, dangerous viruses, including COVID-19.

During my tenure, we knew that pandemic research was a priority. Although our pandemic response plan would be shelved, thankfully, all throughout the coming years, the NIH would fund research into all sorts of pandemic threats, including SARS and the Middle East respiratory syndrome coronaviruses. As a result of decades of research, the NIH would be instrumental in helping a COVID-19 vaccine be developed at an unprecedented speed.

~

It wouldn't be SARS or the H5N1 flu that created one of the greatest challenges in my tenure. Instead, it would be a conflict-of-interest crisis. In 2003, investigative reporting by Pulitzer Prize–winning journalist David Willman of the *Los Angeles Times* accused the NIH of having rampant conflicts of interest. Willman cited specific scientists and payments that, in some cases, over years, added up to hundreds of thousands of dollars.[5] The group of scientists in question were the intramural, or in-house, ones.

"Dual roles—federal research leader and drug company consultant—are increasingly common at the NIH, an agency once known for independent scientific inquiry on behalf of a single client: the public," Willman wrote.[6]

The reporting by the *Los Angeles Times* conveyed a conflict-of-interest crisis shrouded by flawed NIH codes of conduct, as consulting contracts were kept in the darkness and out of the public eye.[7]

I was shocked by the reporting. In becoming director, I'd divested all company shares that could compromise my ability to faithfully serve the American people. I'd followed the rules consistently, regardless of the toll on my personal finances.

I discussed Willman's accusations with my staff. Unbeknownst to me, some scientists could moonlight outside the NIH and not have to fully inform the agency about what they were doing after work hours. The nature of one's work and compensation could be left in the dark. Preexisting, more stringent moonlighting rules had been relaxed before my arrival as director.

The NIH had been losing top scientists because their government salaries were a fraction of what they could earn in academia or industry.

Loosening agency restrictions had supposedly kept them from jumping ship. For the NIH to maintain its supremacy, it needed to keep attracting premier scientists.

Representative Jim Greenwood, who was chair of the House Energy and Commerce Committee's Subcommittee on Oversight and Investigations, wanted all outside consulting activities by NIH scientists to be declared. The NIH was asked to provide records of intramural scientist consulting contracts dating back to 1999.[8] We cooperated with Congress as best we could. I wanted to get to the bottom of this as much as they did. My goal was to navigate this crisis with transparency.

I communicated a clear plan to investigators that included the creation of an expert, blue-ribbon panel composed of individuals from outside the NIH who would offer counsel on the agency's conflict-of-interest rules. Within the NIH, an ethics advisory committee would be established, and the agency would examine employee-received pay from outside sources.[9]

In a letter to Congress that outlined this plan of attack, I also stated, "Our [NIH] mission is too important to the public health of the Nation to have it undermined by any real or perceived conflicts of interest."[10]

After reviewing moonlighting information that NIH scientists disclosed, I observed that some reporting anomalies were minor, but in other cases, there were more significant concerns. All in all, however, what I observed was not unreasonable. For example, some scientists gave grand rounds at academic institutions that received NIH grants. This was part of the normal exchange of ideas in science.

I defended the NIH scientists. I felt we shouldn't lock them in. We should let them interact with other scientists in academia and industry. Even still, I also articulated the need for the agency to do better.

"What is being portrayed in the press is not the reality, but that doesn't mean that we couldn't do a better job of managing the conflict issues."[11]

～

Senator Arlen Specter of the HELP Committee was among the angry voices in Congress: "Is there any reason why a governmental [NIH] employee making as much as the vice president should not be required to fill out a public financial disclosure form?"[12]

Regarding the larger crisis, both the House and the Senate were digging into the matter. Congressional investigators didn't believe the NIH was providing them with all the facts.

I didn't have the power to obtain all the answers from all NIH scientists. Jim Greenwood had subpoena powers, however. He subpoenaed pharmaceutical companies. He wanted to know what relationships they had with NIH scientists. I wouldn't hear the results of this inquiry for some time.

Aware that the NIH rules needed reform, as promised in the plan I'd sent to Congress, I created the NIH Blue Ribbon Panel on Conflict of Interest Policies, led by Norm Augustine, chair of the executive committee of Lockheed Martin, and Bruce Alberts, president of the National Academy of Sciences.[13] My good friend Bill Brody had introduced me to Norm, having advised that I get in touch with him. Bill, who was then still president of Hopkins, was someone I'd turned to for guidance during this conflict-of-interest crisis.[14]

The Blue Ribbon Panel was, as NIH documentation stated, tasked with reviewing "the existing laws, regulations, policies, and procedures under which the NIH currently operated regarding real and apparent financial conflict of interest."[15] The panel was also to review "requirements and policies for the reporting of NIH staff's financial interests, including which interests are subject to public disclosure, and what portion of NIH staff file public disclosures."[16] Additionally, the panel was also tasked "with making recommendations for improving existing laws, regulations, policies, and procedures."[17] Eventually, the panel produced a final report that, not surprisingly, advised the NIH to adopt much more stringent and transparent rules.

In May 2004, new reporting about the conflict-of-interest crisis was still being published in the *Los Angeles Times*. While Willman's reporting had taken aim at the NIH, the *Washington Post*'s Rick Weiss lent some support to intramural scientists. I found myself in the middle of dueling coverage.

~

Jim Greenwood called me in for a congressional hearing on May 12. It was one of many oversight hearings I attended throughout the crisis, yet it proved unforgettable. Norm Augustine and Bruce Alberts were also present and slated to testify. We didn't realize we were walking into an ambush. Norm, who would appear before Congress a hundred or more times in his career, would later say it was the most contentious hearing he'd ever experienced.[18]

Jim Greenwood articulated in his opening remarks that "the [Blue Ribbon] panel's work was a useful step, but it is only the first step as the NIH, the Congress and the American public and interested stakeholders sort out the facts and the issues. . . . It is clear from the cases we have reviewed that some NIH scientists are either very close to the line or have crossed the line."[19]

The congressional investigators hadn't told us about the information they'd received from their NIH moonlighting inquiry. In typical Washington fashion, this was a "gotcha" hearing.

In his opening remarks, Jim Greenwood also expressed, "I believe Dr. Zerhouni has been a man of good intentions throughout [this crisis] and I hold him in the highest esteem. He has been earnestly attempting to respond to the committee's concerns and to help us reach a conclusion of this investigation."[20]

On recollecting this hearing years later, these gentler words would, for me, feel like an exception in an otherwise contentious hearing. The congressional investigators were, at times, quite combative, Jim less so than others. The Blue Ribbon report was thoroughly attacked.

"The panel apparently felt compelled to base its recommendation on their misplaced need to excuse the inexcusable," asserted Representative Peter Deutsch.[21]

"I think very serious shortcomings exist within this report and it doesn't give me much confidence that the changes I think need to happen will be made," stated Representative Diana DeGette.[22]

Norm Augustine was shocked. Usually, he wasn't treated like this.

Investigators put on a slideshow with data they'd received regarding NIH scientists and their moonlighting activities. The reports were alarming. Some of it was, in my opinion, criminal. I wanted to review the information Congress had and act on it.

I later returned to the NIH and had a meeting with the agency's scientists. I felt betrayed.

"I was defending you, and I feel like I was stabbed in the back by people who didn't tell me the full story. I can't defend what I don't know, and I cannot address it as head of the agency if I'm left in the dark."

Unfortunately, I couldn't name names from the subpoena that Congress shared with me. Most scientists at the NIH were honest, hadn't crossed the line, and had no idea of what was really going on. The alarming reports presented by Congress had included only a small fraction of the roughly 17,000 intramural scientists at the NIH.

During the meeting, some of the scientists, led by Ezekiel "Zeke" Emmanuel, jeered at me and attacked me directly, saying that I'd behaved like a wimp in front of Congress. Zeke claimed that if the moonlighting was stopped, there would be an exodus of scientists from the NIH given the relatively low salaries the agency provided. The meeting ended, and I felt the pain of having been attacked so viciously from within my own agency.

Reason and, most importantly, trust had left the room, I concluded. I regretted having shown weakness by blaming the NIH intramural community in its totality when the majority were honest and ethical. From then on, I decided that no matter how hurt I felt, I'd never again share my personal feelings in a public conflict and give politically biased individuals an opportunity to score points.

~

As the crisis raged, Secretary Thompson was angry. He told me I needed to clean up my act at the NIH. If I didn't, he'd do it for me. He brought in the general counsel, Alex Azar.

Azar was on the warpath. "We can't tolerate this. We must have a cleaner administration."

The NIH's principal deputy director, Raynard Kington, and deputy director for the intramural research, Michael Gottesman, and I examined the cases that had been given to us by Congress. Of the few dozen scientists they received reports on, there were about 12 who were truly unethically egregious in their actions. I contacted the Office of the Inspector General and asked them to investigate. I told the guilty scientists to cease and desist their wrongful activities immediately.

"I want you to end your outside commitments or else you can't be here. I cannot tolerate this conduct within the NIH. I don't care what the rules are, even in the most lenient interpretation. You've crossed the line."

A few of the guilty scientists resigned rather than undergo a thorough investigation. Others thought they would be defended by their colleagues and stayed.

~

I was between a rock and a hard place. I was being attacked by the NIH scientific community, who were saying that I was not a good director because I was not standing up for them. Yet they had no idea what the worst offenders had done. Meanwhile, I couldn't truly act to solve the situation because Congress was essentially saying they were going to do it for me.

Congress brought some of the worst offenders before Jim Greenwood and his Subcommittee on Oversight and Investigations. A scientist invoked his Fifth Amendment right. A government scientist, paid by taxpayers, was acting like a member of organized crime. It was as if Congress were interviewing Al Capone. It was horrible.

This was a train wreck. In my mind, my number one concern was that if this continued, there would be a complete loss of public trust in the NIH.

With the crisis ongoing, many at the agency were stepping away from me. Some said that I was going to be fired or resign. However, there were also those who stood by me. My staff worked tirelessly, including legislative aide Marc Smolonsky, principal deputy director Raynard Kington, and associate communications director John Burklow.

~

Outside the agency, support from family and colleagues helped me weather the storm. I was grateful for all who supported me—Nadia most of all.

Even still, I was going through hell. It felt lonely at the top. Yet I wasn't going to let it break me. I was going to survive this crisis and clean up the mess. In my mind, the most important objective was making sure the NIH didn't lose the trust of the American people. That would be a lasting nightmare. Accordingly, I needed to right the wrongs.

There is no wrong time to do the right thing. This is a key principle that the conflict-of-interest crisis taught me.

Some NIH scientists didn't want me to do the right thing—not because they were bad people but rather because they didn't realize what had happened and what the right thing to do was. The right thing was implementing tougher yet still reasonable rules, ones aimed at transparency. In doing the right thing, I could face some immediate, painful consequences. However, the thing that truly harmed people was when they delayed the correction of a wrong.

I needed to act now, yet how would I? Many were grandstanding politically rather than trying to solve a real problem in American medicine that had spilled into the NIH: the rising influence of industrial commercial interests on scientists and physicians involved in developing therapies for patients.

While sitting in my office, I glanced at a beautiful picture of a judo match that my daughter, Yasmin, had taken. In judo, your adversary's attack is a gift, not a threat. Their effort becomes your weapon. Rather than resist when they strike, you can back off and let them fall flat on their face.

I realized that in my situation, the only strategy I had was to back off. I needed to let my opponents overstep their bounds.

A large and overbearing set of rules was provided, constructed in part by HHS and the Office of Government Ethics. Many believed these rules were too excessive. Some scientists said they were going to resign.

Now the crisis had been magnified, and it worked in my favor. If I had continued to resist, those who were pushing against me wouldn't have stopped. By stepping out of the way, I allowed both Congress and HHS to overreach despite their well-meaning intentions. It was judo strategy at work.

Now we could get back to equilibrium. I helped progressively push back the rules until we reached something more in line with what the Blue Ribbon Panel had recommended all along.

In response to these rules, again, some NIH scientists said they were going to leave. Colleagues predicted an exodus. I disagreed. Grievances aside, the NIH was a great place for a scientist to be. In the end, to my knowledge, none or very few scientists actually resigned.

The new rules were reasonable. We were implementing a sunshine strategy. We were shining light into every corner to protect the American people. NIH scientists could interact with the outside world of academia and industry, yet research agreements needed our approval; they wouldn't be done in the dark. Even greater disclosure was required for those making critical research decisions.[23]

~

A key part of the strategy for shepherding the NIH through this crisis had been building and maintaining credibility with the chair of the House Energy and Commerce Committee, Texas Republican representative Joe Barton.[24] Barton had played a major role in the conflict-of-interest investigation, and when I'd promised him change, he'd believed me.[25] My strategy—and Barton's own good judgment—had kept him from targeting me and potentially ending my tenure.[26] To Barton's credit, he'd given me a chance to steer the NIH back on course.

The conflict-of-interest crisis, which had lasted years, was now behind us. I'd been attacked from all sides and abandoned by many. Yet in the end, colleagues who had believed I would not survive it ultimately praised my resilience. Many expressed that they were fortunate to have had me in charge during the crisis and that the NIH had gotten out of it with its head held high.

I was able to get back into the good graces of Congress. Some became my defenders. They were happy I'd helped correct course for the NIH.

The conflict-of-interest crisis was both the most negative and the most positive experience I went through as director. Its resolution would be felt far beyond the walls of the agency.

The NIH's new rules were much more stringent and transparent than what academic centers had in place. Senator Chuck Grassley, who believed we had done the right thing in our resolution of the crisis and was concerned about relationships between academics and industry in promoting drugs, called me. He asked if I would be supportive of a "Sunshine Act." I said I would.

Senator Grassley would ultimately coauthor the Physician Payments Sunshine Act, which would become law in 2010, requiring "that detailed information about payments and other 'transfers of value' worth over $10 from manufacturers of drugs, medical devices and biologics to physicians and teaching hospitals be made available to the public."[27]

Sometimes, the trials and setbacks in our lives, while seeming so destructive in the moment, can actually bring about crucial, helpful changes. In nature, destruction can be a precursor to greater growth and strength.

Pioneers and Political Interference   19

The NIH system of peer review was conservative in its nature. We didn't want to award grants that enabled bad science. There needed to be safeguards. Yet this conservative system didn't adequately promote innovative breakthrough science and scientists. Accordingly, some outside the NIH criticized what seemed like an aversion to innovation. I too saw a problem. I had personally experienced this peer review bias toward more established science rather than taking chances on novel, unproven ideas.

Another key NIH funding issue was related to age. Older scientists were receiving more NIH grants than younger ones. Academic institutions were feeding this problem, imposing a rigid, overly long, multiyear pathway one had to follow to become an independent scientist. An individual might not become an independent scientist with independent funding until the age of 42.

Yet when one looked at the history of science, great breakthroughs were often made by far younger scientists who didn't have a preconceived notion of what was possible or impossible. For example, James Watson had been only 26 years old when he co-discovered the structure of DNA. Tragically, the young men and women who were capable of the next wave of breakthrough science were being stifled by our system.

Accordingly, I championed the creation of the NIH Director's Pioneer Award Program for high-risk, high-reward, breakthrough science. Rather than having a traditional peer review system for these grants, we'd have a jury comprised of scientists with a track record of breakthrough science themselves. It takes one to know one, I felt.

However, I was told this approach would violate the Federal Advisory Committee Act. A solution was suggested by some on my staff: obtain an appropriation waiver from Congress.

To help me in my efforts to obtain this waiver, Ellen Sigal (an influential friend and powerfully effective advocate for cancer research who had made it her mission to accelerate cures for the disease following the tragic loss of her sister) introduced me to Republican senator Ted Stevens of Alaska, who was chair of the Senate Appropriations Committee. Senator Stevens was open-minded and a risk-taker.

We eventually had a meeting in his office. A former pilot in World War II, Stevens was tough. He couldn't be sweet-talked. He reminded me of John Wayne.

"In this Congress, there are workhorses and showhorses. I'm a work-horse," he stated.

Having been a senator since 1968, Stevens knew how Washington operated. He could get things done. Working in my favor was the fact that he loved supporting science. Additionally, during my tenure, the NIH had been good to Alaska, helping its isolated Native American communities to have access to better medical care. I'd personally spent time in the state, getting a sense of conditions on the ground.

Stevens agreed to help me with the pioneer program. I ultimately received the waiver and appropriation language I needed. However, I'd have to create the pioneer initiative as a smaller, pilot program to start. This program would be reviewed after a few years to see if it was worth continuing.

In 2004, nine recipients became the first to receive the award. The brilliant Jeremy Berg (then the director of the National Institute of General Medical Sciences and a former colleague of mine at Hopkins) expressed concern over the reality that "all nine of the first winners [of the pioneer program] were men and about half were already well integrated into the NIH."[1] Although he was not involved in the pioneer program's first year, Jeremy was asked to take the reins for the second year and thereafter to help address the issues he'd raised.[2] His leadership played an invaluable role in the pioneer program's success, just as Senator Stevens had been invaluable in the pioneer program's creation. The accomplished and talented Judith Greenberg would also play a key leadership role in the program.

∼

Among the many notable pioneer awardees, the now Stanford professor of bioengineering and of psychiatry and behavioral sciences Karl Deisseroth would remain in my mind. Part of a new generation of multidisciplinary scientists, Karl combined "bioengineering and psychiatry in studying intact neural circuits in the mammalian brain"[3] and would use "his Pioneer Award to launch a large-scale, systematic effort to map key neural circuit dynamics on the millisecond timescale "[4] He won the award just several years into his thirties. Prior to this milestone, he'd applied for non-pioneer NIH grants and had been turned down.

Into the present, Karl would continue to propel science forward. In 2021, for aiding the development of optogenetics, Karl shared the Lasker Basic Medical Research Award with colleagues.[5] I predict he'll one day receive the Nobel Prize.

Among other pioneer awardees, I was particularly proud of the female scientists we supported. I admired the quality of their work and the strength of their resolve in overcoming barriers of prejudice in their field. Rosalind A. Segal, Karla Kirkegaard, and Rebecca W. Heald were just some of the exceptional scientists we had the privilege of supporting. Similarly, the pioneer program backed some brilliant scientists from ethnically diverse backgrounds, such as the Chinese-born Sunney Xie and the Ghana-born Kwabena A. Boahen.

Eventually, the National Academy of Medicine would review the pioneer program, declaring it to be one of the best components of the NIH Roadmap.

Under the umbrella of the high-risk, high-reward research supported by the roadmap's common fund, the NIH Director's Pioneer Award would be joined by the NIH Director's New Innovator Award, established in 2007. Jeremy Berg and Judith Greenberg spearheaded the conception and development of this new award.[6] It would be intended to support even younger scientists who were budding pioneers rather than full-blown ones. After my tenure ended, even more programs would be added into the high-risk, high-reward research initiative.

For young people out there, you don't have to wait to be 50 to come up with cutting-edge ideas. Youth has its own wisdom, often free of the pessimism and rigidity that can cripple the imagination of the old. Work hard and exercise the patience and persistence needed to make your contributions today, not tomorrow.

The NIH's mission is sacred. The agency must be at the service of all Americans. No disease can be off-limits. Disease knows no politics.

This phrase, which I'd spoken during my confirmation hearing, continued to be my guiding star. As director, I had to keep the NIH from being swayed by anything but science, truth, and serving the American people. This wasn't always easy, as I was working in the rabid world of Washington, with its numerous special interest groups.

Evangelicals and other religious conservatives were among those who tried to influence the NIH.[7] They were an effective faction within the Republican Party, and they had access to the president.[8]

In looking back at my NIH tenure, my legislative aide, Marc Smolonsky, would one day recall,

> Elias had to walk a fine line. If he leaned toward this [religious] faction publicly, he would lose NIH and the scientific community. If he dismissed the religious conservatives, he would lose the support of the White House. He negotiated this difficult path with transparency, honesty, and openness. He maintained credibility with all sides. Had he not, stem cell research would have been outright banned during his time at NIH.[9]

The line was easier to walk some days than others, and I had to learn to do it on the fly. I hadn't stepped into the shoes of NIH director as a seasoned politician.

In one example of religious conservatives trying to influence agency policy, the powerful Traditional Values Coalition (TVC) had philosophical issues with some of the relatively minor grants that the NIH was funding, which included research on HIV and sexuality. The TVC had been established in 1980 by Louis Philip Sheldon, a pastor and "lobbyist for the Lord"[10] with a ferociously anti-LGBTQ agenda. His daughter, Andrea Sheldon Lafferty, the executive director of the TVC, wanted to meet with me, claiming that we were funding "smarmy" grants and should stop.

I refused to meet with her. I wasn't going to get the NIH mixed up in politics. No one group of Americans should be prevented from benefiting from the medical research the agency was tasked to provide.

After refusing to meet with Andrea Lafferty, I received calls from some, trying to push me to change course. It was suggested that there was, perhaps, a happy medium of compromise that I could reach with her regarding the funding of certain grants. Yet in my mind, there was no happy medium.

"The NIH has a peer review mechanism by which it gives research grants, and the TVC isn't going to interfere with it," I responded.

A list of nearly 200 "questionable" NIH-funded or -approved projects was provided to the House Committee on Energy and Commerce by the TVC.[11] Democratic representative Henry Waxman alleged that members of HHS helped put together the list, which was born from confidential information and should not have been given out.[12] Topics on the list included HIV/AIDS prevention, pregnancy prevention, and mental health, and the principal investigators for these projects had their names listed.[13]

In the case of the list, Judith Auerbach of the American Foundation for AIDS Research rightly asserted, "Anything that identifies or targets individual investigators because of the subject matter of their research is unacceptable."[14]

A key Republican congressman who'd been given the list tore into me. He told me that the NIH was misusing public funds. He wasn't the only member of Congress to be upset by what they saw. I soon received numerous letters from both Republicans and Democrats.

When it came to the list of grants that had caused such an uproar, I took time to personally review each one. I confirmed that all the grants were important projects for the NIH to support. One study was about preventing HIV in foster children.[15] Another subject of research was the role of so-called lot lizards in spreading HIV. Lot lizards were prostitutes that worked at trucker rest stops. It turned out that truckers and trucking stops were identified as a major path of HIV spread. Andrea Lafferty claimed these grants were a waste of tax dollars.[16]

I had my staff develop a justification for every grant, explaining why they were important to public health. I was compelled to communicate with Congress, and I would inform them that there was nothing improper with these grants.

I personally drafted a detailed letter that I sent to all members of Congress, including eight key leaders, among them the chair of the House Committee on Energy and Commerce, Republican Billy Tauzin.[17] The letter explained the grants and their importance to public health, detailed the NIH peer review process, and included an attached, six-page summary that gave compelling explanations for all the controversial grants, including the aforementioned topic of lot lizards and HIV transmission.[18]

My letters worked. Members thanked me for explaining the grants. Now they understood the rationale behind them.

My friend and ally Ted Kennedy wrote me, commending my efforts, "If we refuse to allow NIH research to be conducted in areas of medical need because of political considerations, we will do a tragic disservice to millions of patients and their families who count on NIH to explore every possible avenue to improve the prevention, treatment, and cure of disease."[19]

I requested a congressional hearing to go through the grants so that the reasons behind them would be made even more abundantly clear. At the hearing, I gave the needed explanations and articulated that the grants, while focused on certain groups, including transgendered Native Americans, affected each and every one of us. This research served both the few and the many.

Ultimately, the "smarmy" grants crisis was averted. Through this experience, I observed firsthand how politically motivated advocacy groups could influence both the executive branch and Congress. If the TVC had gotten its way, it would have damaged the NIH's credibility and ability to do the research that was needed for the American people. In a larger sense, canceling the grants would have been disastrous for the integrity of science in our country.

I would find out later that it was the White House that had told some of the objectors to back off. I was appreciative of President Bush's support.

During the crisis, we'd spoken privately. I'd let him know the stand I was going take and had offered to resign if my actions would cause too much political heat.

Bush had replied, "Big E, you serve me best by being the best agency head you can be. Don't worry about the heat, I can take it."

～

As director, I contended with groups other than the TVC that aimed to use the NIH to achieve their own objectives. One instance was related to my authority to sign off on a special research waiver that would allow a scientist to study a crime, its causes, and its perpetrators (a unique authority given to the NIH director by Congress). To help understand and prevent evil acts, the NIH studied those convicted of crimes.

Prisoners and their lawyers consented to the research as long as information shared with scientists could not be accessed by the Justice Department. The special waiver allowed me to authorize research along these lines. However, the waiver wasn't something I signed off on frequently. It was used sparingly and only after a rigorous review of the potential project in question.

In the aftermath of the Catholic Church being besieged by allegations of pedophilia, a law firm that was representing the church asked to see me. They wanted to better understand what the drivers and root causes of pedophilia in the priesthood were. They requested that I provide what I saw as a "blanket" waiver, covering the scientific studies that they wanted to undertake, which included interviewing priests and examining their medical records.

If I signed off on the waiver, the problem I saw, as pointed out by the NIH's general counsel, was that every single case the firm accessed for their study could essentially become unusable in the court of law. I didn't want to potentially interfere with the process of justice, as the cases in question involved individuals who had yet to be convicted. As a result, I refused to authorize the waiver.

~

There were times during my tenure when I had to contend with attacks from members of Congress. My encounter with then Republican Speaker of the House Dennis Hastert would stick with me. At the time, Hastert was one of the most powerful men in Washington. Yet his career would ultimately fall apart, and by April 2016, in connection with the sexual abuse of high school children, Hastert would be sentenced to 15 months of federal prison.[20]

Long before this happened, however, during my tenure as director, I learned that Hastert was mad at me. He believed that the appropriations bill he'd lost a vote for had been defeated because of NIH lobbyists.[21] This wasn't true, but regardless, Hastert had a bone to pick with me and the agency.

I went to Hastert's office, accompanied by Marc Smolonsky (my legislative aide), as well as Republican representative Ralph Regula, who played a key role in NIH appropriations. We met with Hastert and his staff.

A former wrestler, Hastert was imposing, almost scary. He was the third most powerful person in the country. We shook hands. It felt like his was twice the size of mine.

"Well, Dr. Zerhouni. I'm so happy to see you. You're finally gracing my office with your presence," Hastert said, dripping with sarcasm.

"What do you mean?"

"People usually come and visit me much sooner when they have an important role like yours."

Earlier in my tenure, I'd tried to meet with Hastert in his district, yet he had canceled on me. I informed him of this.

"Really?" he replied, unsure if it was true.

"Well, ask your staff."

His staff nodded. I was correct.

"Oh, okay," Hastert said. "Well, that's not the issue. The issue is that you influenced the budget vote that I lost by giving the names of some of your buildings to legislators."

Confused, I asked which buildings he was talking about. Hastert mentioned two. I realized that he was referring to buildings at the CDC in Atlanta. He thought they were at the NIH. I made him aware of his mistake.

"Are you sure?" he asked.

"Yes. I'm 100 percent sure."

The meeting would end, but not before Hastert asked me to keep him informed about all the money the NIH was receiving. He wanted to get an update about what the NIH was doing for the American people. His words were threatening.

"I'll certainly do that, sir," I responded. "I hope you'll give me the time and not cancel again."

I prepared a deck of slides for my next meeting with Hastert. It would show the effect the NIH was having on public health and all the key scientific discoveries that had been made, among other agency accomplishments.

Time went by, and I eventually went back to Hastert's office for the next meeting. Marc Smolonsky and Ralph Regula were again with me. From the start, Hastert was aggressive.

"I have a problem with giving so much money to the NIH. I don't know what the American people are getting from your work."

Hastert's attacks persisted. He didn't seem to have any interest in listening to me. Finally, I'd had enough. I wasn't going to be bullied. I took the deck of slides and slapped them on the table.

"I came here to brief you, yet you won't even listen," I said angrily. "You're making your judgments about NIH without considering the data I brought." I lifted up a slide from the deck and showed it to him. "Look at this. It shows that half the hospital beds in the country would be filled with HIV-infected patients if it wasn't for the NIH." I then showed him another slide. "There would be more than a million more people dead from heart disease if we hadn't done the research we did and the treatments we came up with."

I went on, simultaneously making my case for the NIH and pushing back against the third most powerful person in Washington. If Hastert wanted, he could've destroyed me in a millisecond. Ralph Regula was looking at me like I was crazy. Hastert's staff were speechless. Marc Smolonsky tried to get me to calm down. I refused. Ultimately, Hastert backed off, taking a more diplomatic tone.

"I'm just trying to understand what the NIH is doing, doctor."

I proceeded to properly go through the full deck of slides, now in a calmer state of mind. I asserted that the NIH was the crown jewel of the federal government. It saved more lives than any other agency.

It was clear that the meeting had taken a turn for the better. Having listened, Hastert seemed to better understand the value of what the NIH was doing.

"Doctor, I appreciate you coming back and explaining this all to me. You have my support."

At the end of the meeting, we shook hands, and I said I would come back and brief him anytime he wanted.

In the aftermath of the meeting, I learned that what had happened between Hastert and me was spreading around Washington. People were talking about how the director of the NIH had yelled at the Speaker of the House and that the latter had backed off. The episode earned me respect that would be helpful later when the NIH Reform Act needed to reach the finish line.

My encounter with Hastert further framed me as a politically independent figure in Washington. I'd asserted this independence before, yet because I was appointed by a Republican administration, there were some, especially in the scientific community, who likely doubted whether I was truly impartial and apolitical (as I promised I would always be). Disease knows no politics.

Decades later, in recalling the battle between Hastert and me, Marc Smolonsky would say, "If Elias had not turned Hastert around . . . NIH would have lost the goodwill of Congress, and the agency's resources would have been slashed."[22]

The Reform Act, Stem Cells, the French, and Cruising to the Finish Line

20

In 1944, Congress passed the Public Health Service Act, which laid the foundation for a modern NIH, supporting biomedical research through extramural grants, largely to academic research institutions.[1] This basic system remained in place during my tenure and had served the nation well, yet the demands of a new century required the NIH to be reformed with the roadmap for medical research in mind.[2]

Congress had witnessed a successful pilot experiment on how the NIH could be better run with the roadmap. Proper legislative reform could enable the roadmap's aims to be fully realized while ensuring that the initiative would last beyond my tenure. Conversely, without any reform, I'd ultimately lack the means and the mechanism to fulfill my vision as director and serve the American people.

The reauthorization bill that would provide the needed reform was initiated in the House of Representatives by the newly appointed chair of the House Energy and Commerce Committee, Joe Barton, a Republican from Texas. Like me, Barton wanted the reauthorization and reform to happen. It had been more than a decade since the NIH had been reauthorized. I worked tirelessly with Barton and his staff (especially the gifted Cheryl Jaeger) on putting together what would be known as the NIH Reform Act.

Regarding the reform that was needed, I told Barton, "The institutes are strong, but there's not enough coordination between them. The NIH is like a hand with 27 fingers and no palm."

To help make my point, I drew the many-fingered hand for Barton.

Barton laughed, liking my explanation. "So how do we make the palm stronger?" he asked in his Southern drawl.

The answer to Barton's question was a common fund that was far larger and had its funds drawn directly from the government rather than from the institutes and centers.

As we continued to work on the bill, we dealt with the machinations of legislation: lobbyists being for or against it, lobbyists disagreeing with this and disagreeing with that—the obstacles were frequent. The journey would take several years and countless hearings. I now, however, had enough credibility in Washington to be listened to and trusted.

I testified and presented to Barton's committee. I brought along a slide of a little sculpture of a hand with 27 fingers and no palm to help illustrate the same metaphor I'd articulated to Barton. It worked. Eventually, in September 2006, the Republican-majority House approved the bill by a vote of 414 to 2. Partisan politics were cast aside in favor of a greater good and fighting disease.

Yet the Reform Act still needed to be passed in the Republican-majority Senate. To complicate matters, the congressional elections of November 2006 were favorable to the Democrats, who would take over both the House and the Senate in early January. If the bill wasn't passed before the current Congress adjourned, we would have to start all over when the next Congress convened, a setback that would be detrimental to the NIH and the American people.

The clock continued to tick, and the Reform Act stalled in the Senate. I knew we were running out of time. The current Congress would soon adjourn. It seemed like all hope was lost.

"Is there anything that can be done?" I asked Marc Smolonsky.[3]

"Probably not, but if anyone can breathe life into the legislation, it would be Senator Kennedy."[4]

Soon, with Capitol Hill seemingly empty, Marc and I paid Ted Kennedy a visit during which his top staff were present.[5] I made it clear to the senator that I could not achieve desirable and durable changes at the NIH without the reform bill being passed.[6]

"If this bill doesn't pass now, I'm resigning in January. It's my legacy that's on the line. This is what I've worked to achieve for the past four years."

Concerned, Kennedy studied me. "It means that much?"

"Yes."

As we talked, Kennedy's staff were shaking their heads. They said there was no way the bill could be passed in time. They felt the Democrats would be opposed to it.

"Why?" I asked.

"Because they want to put their fingers in it once they get power over the House and Senate. So they want to delay it to January," the staff responded. "Do you understand?"

"I understand, but it's not the right thing to do. It's a disservice to the country."

"Well, Dr. Zerhouni, this is the way Congress works. We can't change that."

Meanwhile, Senator Kennedy had a little smile on his face, the wheels turning in his mind. At the end of the discussion, however, he graciously turned me down.[7] I unhappily began heading to the door, disappointment on my face.[8]

"Wait a minute," Kennedy said.[9] He rubbed his chin and then added, "What the hell. Let's do it."[10]

~

Democratic senators Barbara Mikulski and Patty Murray had indicated they would not approve the bill until the Democrats were in control and it had been reexamined. Kennedy soon spoke with them. Mikulski, who knew and respected me, was persuaded to be on board. Murray, however, wouldn't commit.

"We need to get the SCHIP [State Children's Health Insurance Program] bill passed and the Republicans are blocking me on it," Murray informed Kennedy. "If they want the NIH bill to go through, they'll have to give me this."

The next day, Kennedy called me and said, "You have a chance. But you've got to get the Republicans to agree to what Murray wants."

I went back to Joe Barton and filled him in on what the Democrats were after. Next, I spoke to Democratic representative John Dingell, a giant of a legislator with whom I had a good relationship. Dingell had supported the Reform Act bill. I told him the problem we were facing.

"Let me handle it," he assured me.

Finding a resolution and a version of the NIH Reform Act that could be passed was no easy task, however. The time continued to tick away. Congress's last day before adjourning arrived. The bill had yet to be passed.

By 6 p.m., an agreement still hadn't been reached. I finished my day at the NIH and then spoke to Marc Smolonsky.

He sadly informed me, "Doctor, I'm sorry, but your initiative is dead. There's no way they're going to pass it before midnight."

Heartbroken, I wasn't giving up hope. I went home and put on C-SPAN to monitor what was happening with the bill. It wasn't looking good.

Around 10:30 p.m., I received a call from Senator Kennedy. He was pleased.

"I think we have it. We found a way, and I think you'll be happy. But I want you to stay at NIH. If this passes, you're not moving."

I was in disbelief. "If it passes, I'm not moving, senator."

"You're doing a good job. I want you to be proud because there's a lot of support for what you're advocating. And the naysayers, they're not really a factor here. Dingell, Barton, Murray, Enzi, and I reached an agreement regarding SCHIP. It will be included in the NIH bill. We're just checking the language."

We ended our call. The clock ticked toward midnight. At 11:45 p.m., with the bill still not passed, I was nervous. We were out of time—or so I thought. Soon, I was informed of a motion to extend the legislative session.

Marc Smolonsky called me and said, "When they do this, it means there are last-minute bills that they are reconciling, and they want to get them through. I hope yours is one."[11]

In time, I received another call from Senator Kennedy.

"Watch the TV. Your bill is going to get through."

Right before the end of the congressional session, Chairman Barton brought forward the Senate-amended bill (which had passed the Senate unanimously) for a vote in the House, leading to an overwhelming voice vote and passage. The last item on the bill was about SCHIP. To this day, I'm still asked how that item made it onto the Reform Act.

The next day, I received loads of e-mails. People were shocked. They wanted to know how we had pulled it off. It was persistence, positive relationships in Congress, and the efforts of congressional leaders, among other factors. Joe Barton had tirelessly fought for the Reform Act, and, once again, Ted Kennedy had proved himself a great legislator, helping to usher in a bipartisan victory in the Senate. John Dingell and Republican senator Mike Enzi were among other members of Congress who'd helped the bill succeed.

At the White House, President Bush signed the bill into law. He was quite happy.

"I'm really proud of you, Big E," the president said to me. "You make things happen."

We had made it happen. This was bipartisanship at its best. Public servants on both sides of the aisle had come together to serve the people.

In the politically polarized present, I wish our nation could put aside differences more often and do the same. When it comes to the treatment of disease, it's essential that we cast politics aside.

The Reform Act preserved the core authorities of the NIH while adding new tools to maximize the agency's effectiveness.[12] The new common fund would be colossal compared to what I'd had before. Collectively, for fiscal years 2007 and 2008, I was given $981.2 million,[13] allocated directly from the government, thanks in part to the generosity and vision of Democratic representative David Obey of the appropriations committee.

With this new common fund, no longer drawn from the institutes, I had more freedom in terms of what I could do. I would use it to support high-risk and potentially high-reward, crosscutting, innovative research that no single institute or center could accomplish alone.[14] Research supported by the common fund aimed to fill vital gaps in our knowledge of human biology and allow NIH to be nimble and more responsive to emerging issues and opportunities.[15] Common fund projects included the Human Microbiome Project, with the mission of generating resources enabling comprehensive characterization of the human microbiota and analysis of its role in human health and disease.[16] Another key project was the Structural Biology Roadmap, a strategic effort to create a comprehensive gallery of the three-dimensional shapes of proteins in the body.[17]

With the Reform Act passed, there were now plenty in Washington who felt I was an effective director. I didn't have to prove myself anymore. The White House was supportive, as were key congressional figures. Congress was no longer questioning what the NIH was doing with all its money. The agency had been reauthorized, and there was a renewed period of trust and respect for it. The current secretary of HHS, Michael Leavitt, commented favorably on what had been accomplished.

I found this next part of my tenure, between 2006 and 2008, to be a much smoother ride than earlier years. During this quieter period, I tried to address some of the agency's fundamental problems. One of them was the peer review process, which was in need of reform.

In 2007, with this goal in mind, an internal working group and an external working group were put together. They were tasked with reviewing the NIH peer review process. Each group was cochaired by the gifted Lawrence ("Larry") Tabak, director of the National Institute of Dental and

Craniofacial Research (who would one day serve as the acting NIH director and would eventually retire from the agency and his position as NIH principal deputy director in 2025). The respected and accomplished director of the National Institute of General Medical Sciences, Jeremy Berg, cochaired the internal group and worked closely with Larry.[18] Colleagues started referring to the Larry Tabak and Jeremy Berg duo as "Ta-Berg."[19]

"Ta-Berg" guided the working groups as they drew input from the scientific community. Similar to the construction of the NIH roadmap, we were gathering data from our peers to help properly direct our efforts and reforms. In the end, our final plan aimed for major reform. In June 2008, I announced the coming changes.

As stated in a key NIH press release, the Implementation Plan Report included four priority areas: "engaging the best reviewers, improving quality and transparency of reviews, ensuring balanced and fair reviews across scientific fields and career stages, and developing a permanent process for continuous review of peer review."[20] Also articulated in the press release: when it came to "ensuring balanced and fair reviews across scientific fields and career stages," supporting "a minimum number of early stage investigators and investigators new to NIH" was key, as was continuing "the commitment of—and possibly expand(ing) the use of—the Pioneer, EUREKA, and New Innovator Awards."[21]

Since the beginning of my tenure, one of my persistent worries had been the need to properly motivate and fund the next generation of scientists. Data had showed insufficient funding of young investigators despite the creation of special grant programs designed for them. Meanwhile, demographic analysis had made it clear that we would face an increasingly aged scientific workforce.

After Hurricane Katrina reduced our budget by 1 percent, we were surprised to see that grants to young investigators dropped by 30 percent that year after conventional peer review. This led the NIH to promulgate a different review that ensured that young investigators competed with other young investigators rather than more senior researchers. We established mechanisms to allow postdoctoral fellows to apply, which had not been possible before, and carefully tracked the data. This effort partly stabilized the issue of funding young investigators and was continued by Francis Collins, my successor as director.

∼

By 2007, the embryonic stem cell conflict had reduced in intensity. Japan's Dr. Shinya Yamanaka (who was affiliated with the Gladstone Institute in San Francisco and was a professor at Kyoto University) had, through experimenting with the skin cells of mice, found a way to create induced pluripotent stem cells, born from a process by which mature cells were brought back to an immature state.[22] Yamanaka would receive the Nobel Prize in 2012 "for the discovery that mature cells can be reprogrammed to become pluripotent."[23]

In the United States, President Bush had remained supportive of alternative stem cell research, and, accordingly, the possibility of "reprogramming adult cells to behave as stem cells"[24] had been a welcome development. As a Bush aide would later articulate, this breakthrough replicated "the medical promise of embryonic stem cells without the moral controversy."[25]

Meanwhile, some members of the scientific community still felt that limiting federal funding to the existing 78 embryonic cell lines (many were corrupted or compromised) was unacceptable.[26] Although I knew President Bush's policy toward stem cell research had been a step in the right direction (it had, for the first time, opened federal funding for this research field), I also knew we would need to do more. Expanded research could lead to crucial treatments for diseases.

In the spring of 2007, a Senate panel inquired as to whether I thought the president's stem cell research ban was obstructing the discovery of medical breakthroughs.[27]

I replied, "The answer is yes. It is very clear from my point of view that the current cell lines will not be sufficient to do [all] the research we want to do."[28]

Many were surprised that I would publicly disagree with the president, who had appointed me. Conservative political appointees tried to push me to walk back my statements, threatening to go to the president. I held my ground, willing to resign rather than give in. I also hoped that President Bush would support my political independence. He did.

While I didn't agree with President Bush's decision to later veto legislation that would counter his stem cell research ban, I respected that he didn't punish me for giving my scientific opinion and disagreeing with his administration. Yet again, President Bush had helped preserve the political independence of the NIH.

Meanwhile, his vigorous support for alternative stem cell research would only expand. An Executive Order issued in the summer of 2007 yielded an impactful, increased commitment to studying pluripotent stem cells.[29] The NIH implemented President Bush's call to action with a plan that included "two fresh funding streams to stimulate research on human pluripotent stem cells derived from non-embryonic sources."[30]

The President's Executive Order, among other mandates, had "invited scientists to work with the NIH to add new ethically derived, human pluripotent stem cell lines to the list of those eligible for federal funding."[31] President Bush and the NIH's commitment to pluripotent stem cell research would yield benefits for the American people, underscoring the president's commitment to helping our citizens in a way that he felt was morally acceptable.

$\sim$

When I had assumed my role as director, there was a huge conflict between the NIH and the Pasteur Institute in France (a private foundation tasked with helping treat and prevent diseases through public health initiatives, teaching, and research) connected to the discovery of HIV. In 1983, Pasteur's Francoise Barre-Sinoussi and Luc Montagnier (who would share the Nobel Prize for their discovery of HIV) and their team had published their discovery of the virus. In 1984, the NIH's Robert Gallo and his team had also published their discovery of the virus. The viruses used by these parties were of the same origin. A sample of Montagnier and Barre-Sinoussi's virus had been used by Gallo's lab, though Gallo claimed it was an accident.[32]

As an eventual by-product of Gallo's discovery, at the NIH, an HIV-antibody test was created. With significant profit at stake, Pasteur and the NIH butted heads in regard to whom the patent should belong to.[33] In 1987, French prime minister Jacques Chirac and President Reagan signed an agreement that would result in shared patent royalties for the HIV blood test.[34]

During his tenure (1993–1999), NIH director Harold Varmus took major steps to further resolve the conflict and heal the wounds. The NIH openly acknowledged that NIH scientists had invented an HIV test with a virus from Pasteur, and a new agreement yielded a revised royalty split (for the test kit) more favorable to the French.[35] For test kits sold in France, Pasteur would still pocket the initial 20 percent of royalties.[36] Meanwhile, for test kits sold in the United States, the NIH would still pocket the initial 20 percent of royalties.[37] The collective royalties that remained would be divided up favorably to Pasteur, as they would receive 50 percent, while the NIH received only 25 percent.[38]

Later, during my tenure, the director of Pasteur, Philippe Kourilsky (whose tenure had begun in 2000), came to see me and was aggressive. Despite the changes that had been made, he felt that the NIH owed Pasteur additional royalties for the HIV test. I didn't agree, nor did I appreciate his combative tone. The dispute remained unresolved, and it affected the relationship between the U.S. government and that of France.

Eventually, I received a visit from the new director of Pasteur, Alice Dautry, who had started her role in 2005 and was the first woman to lead the institute. She was intelligent, kind, and not confrontational. We connected and began working toward ending the dispute in a way that would benefit both the NIH and Pasteur. My fluency in French and understanding of the culture helped the discussions move along in a positive direction. Eventually, we came up with a solution that both sides were happy with.

The French ambassador in Washington, Jean-David Levitte, who was quite influential, appreciated what we had accomplished. Ambassador Levitte told President Chirac that they needed to award me the Legion of Honour, as I had helped save the relationship between the NIH and Pasteur. Chirac agreed. In time, I learned that I was to be granted this extraordinary decoration, which had been given before to the likes of scientists like the humanitarian Dr. Jean W. Pape and the courageous, former surgeon general Dr. C. Everett Koop. It was an honor, one that I would not formally receive until after I'd stepped down as director.

In 2007, Nicolas Sarkozy became president of France. Ambassador Levitte became his senior diplomatic adviser. Sarkozy expressed concern about the evolution of biomedical research and development in his country. Levitte spoke to their science adviser, Arnold Munnich, telling him to go see me and find out if I would help them do an evaluation of their National Institute for Health and Medical Research (Inserm).

Arnold visited me at the NIH. He asked me to chair a panel that would handle the evaluation. I was happy to do it and was able to get the permission needed to move forward.

"This panel has to be independent, not beholden to special interests in France," I told Arnold. "The second condition is that the president doesn't have to take our recommendation, but he must say yes or no. Not maybe." It was the same sentiment I'd articulated when Rick Klausner had wanted me to work with the NCI years prior. "And then in terms of membership on the panel, I will have a say on that. I will have a right to approve."

Arnold agreed to my conditions. The French government sent me potential names for the panel, all French scientists. I called Arnold to express my thoughts. The list they had given me felt imbalanced.

I assembled a more appropriate one that we would move forward with. Nobel laureates Harold Varmus, Jules Hoffman, and Peter Agre were part of an impressive, international panel of scientists. One of these brilliant scientists, Jean-Paul Clozel, had left France for Switzerland, frustrated by the system of biomedical research in the former. He was quite skeptical that any change would come from our evaluation

In time, I traveled to Paris, ready to begin evaluating Inserm with my newly assembled panel. I was told that President Sarkozy wanted to meet with us. Before we went to see him, Harold Varmus, who was often casually dressed, preferring T-shirts and jeans to suits and ties, called me.

"Do you have an extra suit that you can loan me, Elias?"

Amused, I loaned him one, and we and the rest of the panel traveled to the Élysée Palace, where the president of France resided. President Sarkozy then met with us.

"I hear you want me to say yes or no when the time comes," Sarkozy said. "For now, I can only assure you that I will take your recommendations very seriously and implement things that are possible to implement."

It wasn't entirely what I wanted to hear, yet I was grateful for President Sarkozy's support. It helped give our panel credibility.

In conducting our evaluation, we used a strategy that I had employed during the development of the NIH roadmap: we connected with the scientific community. We visited labs and interviewed numerous French scientists. In the end, we came up with a helpful, honest report, showing where change was needed. In completing this report, the tireless efforts of Lana Skirboll and Stefano Bertuzzi (a key health science policy analyst at the NIH) were invaluable.

Although we'd been asked to evaluate Inserm, as would be stated in a November 2008 article in *Science*, we made "a diagnosis"[39] and prescribed "a remedy—for the country's [France's] entire biological and medical research sector."[40] Our proposal was honest, and it championed a revamp that would be significant, addressing a flawed, fragmented research enterprise and calling for a unifying agency to emerge.

"This is the first report from a review of the French scientific enterprise that doesn't have the wooden tongue. I love it," Jean-Paul Clozel gushed.

Sarkozy also loved the report. "This is exactly what I want. It's candid. You're telling us what is wrong, what is right, and what we should do. I thank you, Dr. Zerhouni, and I promise you we'll take this seriously."

Although the government was supportive of our report, there was backlash in the French scientific community, including with some union members. Regardless, the president was true to his word. He created a multi-billion-euro program to revamp research and development (R&D) in France.

~

As the fall of 2008 began, the NIH was in good shape. I was cruising, and I realized the finish line wasn't too far ahead. I was ready to move on.

In Washington, directors left agencies under two circumstances. Either they decided to manage their exit themselves, or they were thrown out by the next administration. I decided that I was going to be in control of my exit.

I could leave before the next election or after it. If I waited until after and the Republicans retained the White House, by stepping down, I could be seen as giving up or not supporting the current administration. On the other hand, if the Democrats took control of the White House, they might ask for my resignation letter. Essentially, if I wanted to leave, I ought to do it before the election.

I informed President Bush that I wanted to step down. He was sad to see me go.

"You've done a great job. Why don't you stay, Big E?"

I was firm in my decision. The president granted my request.

Soon, Ted Kennedy also tried to persuade me to stick around. If Barack Obama was elected, Kennedy said he would try to convince him to allow me to stay. I appreciated Kennedy's offer, yet my mind was unchanged.

There was a farewell gathering for me at the NIH. As a humorous yet meaningful parting gift, my staff gave me a jar with rocks, pebbles, and sand inside. They also gave me a little sculpture of a hand with no palm and 27 fingers as well as a list of aphorisms that I'd come up with and always told them, such as that there is no wrong time to do the right thing.

Among the memorable speeches, Tony Fauci, a friend and supportive colleague, delivered a touching farewell, saying, "You arrived as an outsider, and you will leave as one of us, but more than that, a great leader among us."

~

At the end of October, I left the NIH for good and went home. It was a quiet, friendly, no-stress exit. They took my beeper, my phone, and my keys, and I left.

There were stories about individuals in high-profile jobs becoming depressed after leaving them. They were used to having a lot of support and secretaries and things of that sort, and then they found themselves with none of it. No longer in the role of director, I felt relief rather than sadness.

I had done my job, and in the process, I hadn't embarrassed myself too much. For me, life went on.

~

In January 2009, I received a call from the White House. President Bush's second term was coming to a close.

Over the phone, one of Bush's secretaries informed me, "The president wants to thank five members of his administration who he thinks have done an extraordinary job, and you're one of them. Would you please come with your family to the Oval Office on January 19th?"

When the day arrived, my family and I went to the White House. The president was there, and we spent around 45 minutes with him. He expressed his gratitude to me and to my family. President Bush was grateful for the support that Nadia and my children had given me during my tenure.

Before we left the Oval Office, President Bush gave me a handwritten letter of thanks. It was a thoughtful gesture. I enjoyed that his penmanship was as bad as mine.

"Okay," I said to myself. "I'm not the only one with terrible penmanship."

I would remain extraordinarily grateful for all President Bush had done for me and the NIH. For example, there had been moments when some in his administration or Congress had sought to slow down or stop the promised doubling of the NIH budget. I'd reached out and appealed directly to the president, and each time, he'd kept his promise to keep the budget doubling on schedule despite the financial burden of war in the Middle East.

President Bush truly cared for the NIH. He visited the agency five times when I was director, which, as far as I know, is more than any other president before or since. He supported the mission of the agency and its political independence.

~

In a post-9/11 era where anti-Muslim sentiment was common, as director, it was rare that I ever felt discriminated against. The prejudice I did face was veiled rather than overt. In truth, earlier in my career, as a foreign medical graduate and radiologist, I experienced far more discrimination. Yet I didn't let it hold me back no matter how upsetting it was.

Prejudice is an inescapable part of life. Inevitably, you will face it. What matters is that you don't back down because of it. You can't let others define what you are capable of. If I had listened to the doubters at the beginning of my tenure, where would I have ended up? How could I have served the American people?

If you want to lead, you're going to have to put up with doubters—with people who question you, criticize you, and tell you that you will never succeed. As a leader, there's no red carpet that is rolled out for you. You must be ready to weather attacks from all sides, especially when you try to change things.

~

In looking back at my NIH years, there were accomplishments, apart from those that have been mentioned, that stood out. We challenged the obesity epidemic through a major research initiative, we made NIH-funded peer-reviewed research publications available to the public, we made strides in women's health (such as completing a vaccine that would help protect against human papillomavirus, which can cause cancer), and we worked to support female scientists and their careers.[41] The sum total of my tenure, which reflects the tireless efforts and accomplishments of countless dedicated NIH employees, could fill more pages than this book.

When I look back at my legacy, I realize I would have been nothing without those who worked alongside me. It takes a village to achieve, and I have more than a village to thank. I was and always will be grateful to my staff, institute directors, members of the scientific community, members of Congress, the president, and, of course, my loving wife and children, among others. They all played a role in supporting me during these years.

As I arrive at the closing words of part III of my memoir, I want to underscore that the episodes I've described from my NIH tenure are the sum of a whole rather than separate pieces. They reflect a consistent, data- and collaboration-driven management style coupled with a relentless drive for meaningful reform.

MY FUTURE AND PHARMA   IV

Legion of Honour, the Gates Foundation, and Becoming a Presidential Envoy

21

During my NIH tenure, I'd learned I was to be made a Knight of the French Legion of Honour. President Sarkozy invited me and my family and friends to the Élysée Palace. There, he would give me the award. Not every Legion of Honour recipient personally received their medal from the French president. I was fortunate.

At the ceremony, as I sat in the audience, having not yet received the medal, Sarkozy stood at the podium, delivering a kind introductory speech about me.

During it, he looked at me and said, "Elias, I want you to know that your panel's recommendations for our R&D have been put in place. I promised it to you, and I'm doing it."

In France, protocol dictated that no one talked after the president. Accordingly, when the president gave the recipient their medal, the latter was supposed to say thank you and then move on.

Yet when President Sarkozy gave me my medal and we were face-to-face, I asked, "Can I thank you personally and give a little talk?"

He told me I could. I did so, and the people in charge of protocol were horrified. I could see them staring at me as I went ahead and thanked Sarkozy and told him something that I had long since believed in.

"You know, there are two philosophies in life, Mr. President. There's the 'why?' philosophy and the 'why not?' I believe in the 'why not?,' and I think you've done just that in saying, 'Why not push France into the panel's recommendations for R&D?'"

In the audience, among my family, my mother was present. Weeks before the ceremony, when I had informed her that President Sarkozy wanted me to come to the Élysée to receive the medal, she had told me to turn it down.

"Why?" I'd asked.

"In Algeria, during the time of French rule, people who got this medal were usually collaborators. And so, if you get this medal, I won't talk to you again because you'll be a traitor to your country."

"Mom, the war has been over for decades. I mean, what are you talking about?"

I'd tried to convince my mother to change her mind. This award had nothing to do with colonial collaboration. My brothers echoed my sentiments. Eventually, my mother relented and agreed to come to the ceremony at the Élysée.

After it was over, a picture was taken of her with Sarkozy and myself.

My mother spoke with Sarkozy, saying, "It's very kind of you to recognize my son. You know he's Algerian. He's not American. You know that, right?"

"Oh, Madame, I know this," Sarkozy replied. "I know his story very well."

~

Following my departure from the NIH, I was exhausted. I wanted time off. Meanwhile, I was approached by several academic institutions to consider taking their top job.

Hopkins asked me to consider becoming president of the university. Having served as president for more than 12 years, Bill Brody had moved on to new opportunities. His legacy was extraordinary.

A university president was a manager and a leader. Much of it involved fundraising for the institution. I didn't want to go back to living inside a glass bubble like I had during my NIH tenure. Accordingly, I removed myself from consideration for the role.

Hopkins would go on to choose Ron Daniels as its next president. Coupling extraordinary stewardship with bold, impactful initiatives, Ron would support multidisciplinary collaboration, breaking down traditional barriers in academia while also championing Hopkins's commitment to diversity and academic excellence. Hopkins has and always will be my home away from home, and I'm grateful for all that Ron, like Bill Brody before him, has done to better the institution.

Having removed myself from consideration from Hopkins, I knew I wanted to pursue something else, though I didn't know what it was. At the time, I had no intention whatsoever of going into industry, which for academics was the equivalent of going "to the dark side." I was instead considering foundation work. I'd seen the invaluable, life-changing efforts of great philanthropists like Bill Gates and Mike Bloomberg. I wanted to be a part of something like that, something that helped humanity.

Dr. Tachi Yamada reached out to me. Tachi had, in the 1990s, interviewed me at the University of Michigan regarding their opening for radiology chair. During my NIH tenure, I'd appointed Tachi to my advisory council. Tachi was a superb adviser, and, after later going into industry as head of R&D at GlaxoSmithKline (GSK), he was now working with the Gates Foundation. He asked me to become a senior fellow for their Global Health Program.

I accepted the role. Through it, I would "advise the foundation on a range of topics, particularly the Grand Challenges in Global Health initiative."[1] (As mentioned in chapter 17, these grand challenges were significant "scientific challenges that, if solved, could lead to key advances in preventing, treating, and curing the diseases and health conditions contributing most to global health inequity."[2])

I intended to spend half my time, much of it self-directed, working with the foundation. My new boss, Bill Gates, was both brilliant and demanding in the right ways. I was amazed by his passion for the foundation and its mission. For Bill Gates, philanthropy wasn't just about giving out checks. It was about stepping up to actively drive meaningful change and yield tangible results. Mike Bloomberg also operated like this as a great philanthropist for Hopkins and the world.

~

During these years, in addition to taking part in foundation work, I also formed a consulting company, the Zerhouni Group, which would partner with countries, sovereign wealth funds, companies, and institutions that shared my goal of accelerating global innovation by promoting science, technology, and research.

I received a call from Chris Viehbacher, the GSK executive whom I had met during the PEPFAR trip to Africa. Chris had recently been named CEO of Sanofi, a global, French pharmaceutical company headquartered in Paris.

Chris felt I had done an extraordinary job at the NIH. He wanted me to take the reins of Sanofi's struggling R&D organization. I was taken aback. The last thing on my mind was going to work in the pharmaceutical industry. Yet I was somewhat intrigued by the offer, and I suggested that I instead act as a consultant.

"Well, maybe that's the best way to start," Chris replied.

My "cooling off period" post-NIH had ended, meaning that I was now allowed to engage in pharma industry work. I soon began my consulting for Sanofi, but only after I ascertained that Chris had a real strategy for the company's future and was committed to leading with science foremost in mind. He would do so and was brilliant at it. He'd been a member of the board of Research!America, where he'd learned about the entire research enterprise of the United States and the NIH in particular.

As a consultant, my objective was to first complete an in-depth review of Sanofi's R&D organization and offer advice for improvement. Although I knew a great deal about R&D, I didn't know as much about the pharma industry side of it. I'd need to learn fast, and to complicate matters, I didn't have a big team of consultants working with me.

As part of my deep dive into Sanofi's R&D, I did a worldwide tour of their major R&D sites. In the end, I was deeply convinced that the organization needed serious reform. They were betting too much on small-molecule drugs. These drugs, which made up most of the market, had clear advantages. For example, they could penetrate cells with greater ease and be taken orally. Yet small-molecule drugs were also quite difficult to develop, and the hit rate was unbelievably low.

Meanwhile, Sanofi had some great biologics that they weren't developing, which was a huge mistake. Biologics were large-molecule drugs drawn or made from living organisms. Monoclonal antibodies aimed at battling cancer and recombinant human insulin were examples of biologics. Biologics were the rising wave of new medications, partly because they could be developed faster than small-molecule drugs. Unfortunately, a previous Sanofi CEO had been against biologics, and the current state of the company's R&D reflected this.

Sanofi's R&D also struggled because scientists at sites were stopped from publishing their research and exchanging ideas with the larger, outside community. Too much was confidential, and Sanofi's R&D lacked creativity and vision.

I observed that, as an organization, Sanofi was bicephalic. Years prior, the pharma company had acquired Aventis. Aventis was open to biologics, new ideas, and exchanges of information. They had an open strategy, while Sanofi had a closed, secretive strategy.

Consistent with the Aventis merger, Sanofi had grown over the years through acquisitions. It was a conglomerate of multiple companies that had never truly been integrated into one. In a sense, Sanofi didn't have a single R&D organization. It had 31 research sites in multiple countries (only one in the United States). Many sites were, in reality, fronts to show various governments that Sanofi was committed to jobs and R&D in their respective country, thus facilitating access and tax advantages for Sanofi's products. Accordingly, many of these research sites were unproductive.

These separate organizations were not truly growing together. On top of that, Sanofi's R&D was led primarily from Paris by French employees. It didn't have diversity, nor did it have leading-edge scientists in emerging fields. In this R&D conglomerate that lacked integration, the overarching authority from the Paris headquarters was often stifling.

"See this pencil?" a German scientist said, holding it up in front of me. "For me to buy a box of them, I have to get permission from Paris."

∼

The pharmaceutical industry is brutally competitive. The lifespan of pharma companies, excluding the biggest ones, is relatively short. The patent cliff is always looming.

At the end of a drug's patent life or exclusivity, other companies can come in and manufacture generic versions. A company that held a now expired patent can see a 90 percent drop in their product's revenue. As a result, R&D in pharma is a fast-moving treadmill. You must always be searching for the next blockbuster therapeutic. And after you find it, you must start searching for the next one.

Drug development is incredibly expensive. The costs to perform clinical trials and manufacture a molecule into an approved drug are sizable. In pharma, 15 or 20 percent of revenue might go toward R&D. In other industries, at most, it'd be 6 or 7 percent of revenue.

And what if a new drug fails to perform in clinical trials? The success rate for new molecules is unbelievably low.

∼

With patent cliffs looming, the weak state of Sanofi's portfolio didn't bode well for the future. Chris Viehbacher, being the smart CEO he was, knew it.

"Sanofi is going to lose half of its revenues over the next several years. I need to find out if my R&D organization can overcome that or not," he had told me.

After completing my review, I reported my thoughts to Chris and Sanofi's board. I informed them that their R&D organization was not going to deliver unless it was changed. In response, they asked me to formulate a strategic plan. I agreed to do so.

Meanwhile, to save money, Sanofi had decided to close its Boston R&D site. I called Chris and told him this was the absolute opposite of what they should do. Boston was the most important center of biomedical research in the world. Chris intervened right away, taking my advice.

Eventually, I presented a plan for R&D reform to Sanofi's board. They had to reduce their number of R&D sites and integrate the ones they had into more coherent units of research. Regarding the overarching and at times paralyzing authority in Paris, governance reform was needed. Additionally, the overall scientific plan for R&D had to change.

"If you want to have products in the market in time to overcome your patent cliff, you must get into biologics," I insisted. "Developing a monoclonal antibody candidate takes four years, while developing a small-molecule one takes seven years."

Part of the strategy I proposed included partnering with great companies to offset Sanofi's weaknesses. Regarding the current head of Sanofi's R&D, though I personally liked him, the company needed to bring in someone else. I suggested a top replacement candidate whom Chris then tried to recruit. However, this candidate ultimately took a job in academia, leaving Sanofi still in need of a new R&D head.

Soon enough, Chris told me, "We buy into your advice and strategy, and you've been an outstanding consultant. Yet I know you're not a consultant type. You're not going to stay on the sidelines for the rest of your life. You're too young for that. Why not consider taking the job yourself?"

It was an interesting opportunity, though I wasn't sure about my answer—at least not yet.

~

While this era of my life took me into the world of pharma, it also unexpectedly pulled me back into government. President Obama planned to give a global policy speech in Cairo in June 2009 in which he would propose "a new beginning between the United States and Muslims around the world, based upon mutual interest and mutual respect."[3] The stakes for the speech were high. The United States had earned a reputation in the Muslim world and elsewhere of using "hard power," exemplified by the wars in Iraq and Afghanistan. As a result, the United States had lost much of its prestige and trust.

Obama wanted to bring that prestige and trust back and break away from using only hard power. He felt that "soft power" was also important, such as cultural exchanges and exchanges of science and technology. In those days, plenty of lower- to middle-income countries didn't have a science and technology strategy that was driven or at least encouraged by the United States.

In the preparation leading up to Obama's pivotal speech, I unexpectedly received a call from the White House. My name had been given to them by esteemed biochemist and former president of the National Academy of Sciences Bruce Alberts. The White House asked if I would help them with the preparation of Obama's speech. When it came to exchanges of science and technology, the president wanted ideas. Given my scientific background and that I was from Muslim-majority Algeria, they thought I would provide a valuable perspective.

I worked with a team at the White House. Regarding exchanges of science and technology, I advised that they connect Obama's speech with the creation of economic well-being. Helping the well-being of other nations could go a long way in helping to improve the reputation of the United States.

I also suggested that they appoint a few envoys for science and technology who would represent the president. During his speech, the president could talk about the creation of these envoys whom he would send to the different countries we were discussing.

The idea took off. The speechwriters loved it. A portion of the speech was crafted to mention the envoys. When Obama gave the speech in Cairo, that portion was still in there.

"We'll open centers of scientific excellence in Africa, the Middle East, and Southeast Asia, and appoint new science envoys to collaborate on programs that develop new sources of energy, create green jobs, digitize records, clean water, grow new crops."[4]

In time, I received another call from the White House. I was informed that President Obama wanted me to be one of three presidential envoys for science and technology. I was honored to accept the offer. The other two envoys were Bruce Alberts and Nobel laureate Ahmed Zewail. We were named in November 2009.

The President's Council of Advisors on Science and Technology, co-chaired by Harold Varmus, John Holdren, and Eric Lander, had discussed the program and proposed the names of the envoys selected.[5] It is hard to determine who should be credited with establishing the envoy program itself, and I will not try to do so here. For this memoir, my objective is to convey my experiences as an envoy.

As envoys, there were priority nations we needed to visit and establish better scientific and technological ties with; I would cover areas of Europe, the Middle East, and Africa,[6] among them, my homeland of Algeria.

As presidential envoys, we were tasked with helping to build relationships and create new science and technology collaborations in the countries we visited.[7] We were allowed to meet with heads of state.

My travels began. I arrived in Algeria and was received warmly. I'd come a long way since my humble childhood, the days of spearfishing off the coast of Pointe Pescade and struggling with my penmanship in school. Now I was meeting with government leaders and being interviewed on television. However, President Abdelaziz Bouteflika, who knew my family, couldn't meet with me due to how busy he was and health issues.

I traveled to Morocco and met the prime minister there. The government seemed stable and forward-thinking. Morocco wanted to build economic ties with both the United States and Europe. Their strategy was to become a broker between the two.

In Tunisia, I received red-carpet treatment. I met with the ministers of health and higher education as well as the prime minister. Everyone said all the right things. Yet Tunisia was a police state, run by the dictator Zine El Abidine Ben Ali, who would be overthrown in 2011. I was always careful with what I said.

Similarly, during my trip into Muammar Gaddafi's Libya, I also had to speak with caution. After arriving, I met with our ambassador and was briefed. The briefing was in a tent, called a Faraday cage, that was inside our embassy. It was designed to prevent the Libyans from using any listening devices to spy on our conversations.

I left the embassy with our ambassador, and we eventually met with the Libyan minister of education, research, science, and technology. On arriving, I observed that he was frightened.

"Is everything okay?" I asked in Arabic.

He explained that he wasn't sure if the meeting had been approved by Gaddafi.

"I'm sorry," I replied. "We've been requesting this meeting for a while. But if you want, we can leave."

"No, no. Sit down." He responded, still filled with fear.

The meeting proceeded, and the minister barely said a thing. Soon enough, however, he received a call. He excused himself to take it, then returned shortly after smiling wide. He'd been told that our meeting was an approved one. What a stressful way to exist, I thought. I was glad I didn't work for a dictator.

As my trip in Libya progressed, I learned that Gaddafi would not be able to meet with us. However, his son, Saif al-Islam, was available to see us. He was known to be progressive, wanting to open his country up to the world and rebuild its science and technology.

We met with him in the city of Sirte, where his father was from. Gaddafi liked to live in tents, yet Saif al-Islam lived in a house. We sat with Saif al-Islam in a garden. Tea was brought out. Saif al-Islam spoke perfect

English and was accompanied by the Libyan chief of security, the second most powerful man in the country. They had plans to revitalize education and advance science and technology in Libya.

Suddenly, the conversation took a tense turn as Saif al-Islam turned to me and said, with suspicion, "What are you really here for?"

"President Obama wants to establish stronger ties with Libya on the science and technology front to help train the next generation of Libyans and increase employment."

"Is that all?"

"Yes."

My words could not remove his suspicion, yet the meeting continued and concluded well enough. Later, in private, a U.S.-trained Libyan doctor who'd accompanied Saif al-Islam made an unusual request of me.

"Is there any way we can do business with you?"

"What do you mean?"

"We always need to send money into the U.S., to different accounts to be able to pay for Libyan students and other things like that."

I smelled a trap. The doctor was trying to get me to do something illegal. I immediately shut the conversation down, saying that I couldn't help.

It's important to recognize when true dangers arise. Seemingly small decisions that violate legal or ethical foundations and values can destroy one's career. If you're going to survive as a leader, you need to know when to say no.

As an envoy, I visited plenty of countries that were far safer than Libya. In Qatar, it was clear they admired American science and technology and wanted more of it. This was a nation where we had strong ties. They wanted to create their own equivalent of the NIH. I said we would help them. Ultimately, we did.

In India, which I had visited while still NIH director, they were receptive to our mission. I met with government ministers whom I knew. Without delay, Prime Minister Manmohan Singh agreed to meet with me. Singh knew who I was and had visited the NIH. Accordingly, I was received by him far faster than most diplomats, to the chagrin of the U.S. ambassador, who had not been granted a meeting for months and came along with me and my team to share some diplomatic messages.

I found Prime Minister Singh to be kind, thoughtful, and well informed about the health care issues of India, particularly infectious diseases. He clearly believed that disease knew no politics. It was likely why he welcomed us.

I explained to him that I'd come, in part, to ask for his help with facilitating the approval of NIH grants given to meritorious Indian researchers.

The funding was being halted by Indian government ministries that were not giving the needed approvals on time due to arcane rules and long delays. Singh was supportive and willing to help solve the problem. Ultimately, our meeting was productive and a good demonstration of the global soft power of the United States via biomedical research.

As an envoy, I learned that people around the world wanted America to be more predictable. People disliked that U.S. policies, unlike those of other governments, could drastically change every four years. They were more comfortable with forming business relationships with U.S. companies, which they believed were more consistent and predictable than the U.S. government.

Overall, the envoy program was a success. I was grateful to have been a part of it.

～

As I kept myself busy with a number of pursuits, I soon received another call from Tachi Yamada, who had invited me to become a senior fellow at the Gates Foundation.

"Elias, I just got a call from the president and CEO of Danaher, Larry Culp. They are interested in having a life sciences person on their board," Tachi said. "They asked me if I wanted the role, but I told them, 'The best person available, if you act fast, is Zerhouni.'"

Danaher was a massive industrial conglomerate. To give a sense of scale, in 2007, Danaher had bought Tektronix, a test and measurement equipment maker, for $2.85 billion. In the early 1980s, I hadn't even known how to start a company, yet now here I was, decades later, meeting with Danaher CEO Larry Culp. Larry was an articulate, strategic, and transformative leader who'd been named CEO at the young age of 37. He would later become CEO of General Electric and achieve great success.

Larry and the Danaher board were exploring a different strategy going forward. They wanted to move into a steadier industry, and life sciences was something they were considering. I agreed to get involved and joined the board.

I learned as much as I contributed. The board, chaired by Steven Rales (a cofounder of the company with his brother, Mitchell) had three exceptional strengths. First, they operated with a rigorous management approach they'd adopted from using the Toyota methods of continuous and rigorous performance improvement (which, initially, Toyota had learned from the American W. Edwards Deming, industrial engineer and economist, who had been ignored by American companies). Second, the board employed a thorough approach to merging and acquiring other companies that could be improved by Danaher. Third, they used a proactive, strategic approach to how Danaher adapted to the global environment.

Danaher successfully shifted toward life sciences in a period of 10 years. In the present, they are a leading company in the life sciences and technology fields. I'm honored to have been a part of this transformation.

⁓

During this stage of my career, as I engaged in new pursuits, I felt a strong commitment to improve translational research in the United Sates. Direct translation of scientific discoveries into treatments for disease was not the rule.[8] Often, approaches to treatment that worked in vitro or in animal models didn't work in patients.[9] This illustrated the daunting intricacy and diversity of biological systems and the challenge of translational medicine.[10]

Several undercurrents had been rocking biological research, and among them was the uneasy sense that our approach to transforming the past 50 years of advances into better cures, treatments, and preventive measures for disease had not been as effective as it needed to be.[11] At a time of unprecedented opportunities for progress, productivity by pharma and biotech companies had dropped, and there was a growing avoidance of clinical research by promising young scientists.[12]

Knowing that the United States needed more and better translational research, in late 2009, the American Association for the Advancement of Science and *Science* magazine (led by Bruce Alberts) launched *Science Translational Medicine*, of which I was a founding editor.[13] The objective was "to promote human health by providing a forum for communicating the latest research advances from biomedical, translational, and clinical researchers from all established and emerging disciplines relevant to medicine."[14] I hoped the creation of this journal would provide crucial cross-fertilization and synergy among researchers across disciplines, aiding them and paving the way for a future in which more groundbreaking innovations in the diagnosis, prevention, and treatment of disease were realized.[15]

⁓

While pushing to advance translational medicine in the United States, in unrelated work, I managed to consult for a global range of clients in tandem with my stellar team at the Zerhouni Group. This small group of employees included my son, Will, as well as Lana Skirboll, former director of policy at the NIH.

Former congressman Jim Greenwood (a tireless, quite respected public servant who had, during the NIH conflict-of-interest crisis May 12 hearing, confronted me aggressively) reached out to me and the Zerhouni Group on behalf of the Biotechnology Innovation Organization (BIO). BIO was the trade association for more than 1,000 biopharmaceutical companies (BIO represented biotechnology companies, academic institutions, state biotechnology centers, and related organizations across the United States and other countries). Jim was now its president and CEO. He wanted help with developing a plan to improve the policy environment for the innovation of new medicines.[16]

Jim and I put together a long-term strategy that was endorsed by the BIO board and led to significant legislative success for the organization. Jim was grateful. Into the present, we would remain friends.

Aware that he was a bird-watcher, I would one day jokingly tell Jim, "I wish I'd known you were a birdwatcher during the conflict-of-interest hearings. I would've talked to you about birds and softened you up."

~

Despite the many pursuits I engaged in, Chris Viehbacher's offer to become head of Sanofi's R&D remained on my mind. I considered it in depth as I enjoyed a vacation in the Mediterranean. Bruce Holbrook and his wife, Suzie, accompanied Nadia and me on a rented, private boat that departed from Bodrum, Turkey. We were out at sea for days, stopping from time to time at nearby ports.

I still loved to fish, and one day, the Turkish captain and I went spearfishing for octopus. As was the case in my youth, I could still free dive to great depths and hold my breath for long periods. These skills hadn't faded with time, nor had my love of the sea. My son, Adam, would one day say that my diving and swimming had an understated showmanship about it, that I'd navigate the waters with calm and humor. Algerians loved humor, so this made sense.

The Turkish captain and I caught enough octopus for a tasty meal. We cooked them up, and everyone enjoyed them.

During the trip, I discussed with Bruce whether I should shut down my consulting company and take the Sanofi job. Bruce advised me to do so. My mother and three brothers lived in Paris, where the headquarters were located. I missed them, and this opportunity would reunite us to an extent (especially with my mother, to whom I had always been close). Part of Nadia's family also lived in France.

I also liked the idea of taking on a new and daunting challenge. There was an opportunity for me to change things for the better at Sanofi. I could reform a massive R&D organization and help bring groundbreaking new therapies to patients, a dream of many physician scientists. The prospect was exciting. Additionally, Chris offered me the opportunity to maintain my academic positions, including chair of innovation at Collège de France (I'd been elected in 2010). I would, however, have to leave the Zerhouni Group, which meant I would no longer be getting to work closely with my son, Will, an opportunity that I had cherished. I'd also be saying good-bye to some exceptional colleagues, Lana Skirboll included.

Chris called me in December 2010, wanting an answer to his offer. I mulled it over for a little longer. Finally, I called him back and agreed to move forward. I was going to take the plunge. Pharma, quite unexpectedly, was now my future.

Sanofi   22

In January 2011, I became head of global R&D at Sanofi. I stepped onto the treadmill of the pharmaceutical industry. Sanofi's drug portfolio was in a sorry state. Patent cliffs were fast approaching. Chris Viehbacher told me that, by 2015, we needed a new product pipeline that could support the company.

Thankfully, the extensive consulting I'd completed for Sanofi had prepared me for this moment. I was deeply familiar with the R&D organization, and I knew its leaders. I had a vision for how we should move forward.

We didn't have the knowledge or expertise in biologics we needed, so we developed and put in place a three-pronged strategy to address the issue. These were our "rocks." Number one, we were going to partner with companies that were at the leading edge of biologics. Number two, we were going to acquire companies that were at the leading edge of biologics. And number three, we were going to, in time, try to develop our own proprietary biologic platforms to leapfrog the field.

Regarding number two, Chris Viehbacher was looking at companies to acquire. Sanofi eventually decided to acquire Genzyme, a Cambridge, Massachusetts–based biotech company, for $20.1 billion in the second-largest acquisition in biotech history.[1]

Genzyme had difficulties in manufacturing.[2] Sanofi had the manufacturing talent needed to fix these woes. Meanwhile, Genzyme had the talent and innovative biologics that were lacking at Sanofi. In one brilliant move, Sanofi established itself as one of the most prominent pharma companies in Boston, the mecca of pharmaceutical research and development. Genzyme became a key engine that drove growth at Sanofi.

In line with the first part of our three-pronged strategy (partnering with companies that were at the leading edge of biologics), Sanofi reinforced its alliance with the biotech company Regeneron. I'd observed Regeneron's performance and scientific accomplishments from my vantage point at the NIH. A child of immigrants, George Yancopoulos, Regeneron's cofounder (along with Leonard "Len" Schleifer) and chief scientific officer, was brilliant and groundbreaking in his capacity to discover and invent. Meanwhile, CEO Len Schleifer was unusual in his directness and savvy, with a strong and determined personality I liked. Len thought for the long term.

In a time when most companies sought to be bought out by larger ones, Len told me, "I want to make Regeneron the next Genentech and not sell out to anyone."

Regeneron would succeed mightily.

The Regeneron–Sanofi alliance would also succeed. Through it came the biologic dupilumab. Known under the product name Dupixent, this biologic's applications would include eczema and asthma and several other indications. It is now one of the leading drugs worldwide.

The third piece of our three-pronged strategy, trying to develop our own proprietary biologic platforms to leapfrog the field, was also pursued with vigor. We created three laboratories for breakthrough science. One was in France, tasked to find a drug to combat mutated KRAS, an oncogene known to drive the growth of many cancers. Another lab was in Germany, pursuing novel treatments for diabetes and obesity. The third lab was in Boston, built around the concept of multi-specific antibodies directed to diverse targets and vaccines for viral disease and cancer. We wanted to develop "smart molecule" biologics that could attack a disease on multiple fronts. If a disease was multifactorial, why not use a smart, multifunctional biologic molecule to beat it?

In 2012, I recruited Gary Nabel, who'd led the Vaccine Research Center at NIH's NIAID, to become Sanofi's chief scientific officer and head of the Boston breakthrough lab. Gary was a world-class immunologist, virologist, and vaccine expert. Yet another exceptional mind involved in the lab was Zhi-yong Yang (brought on in 2013 as the lab director). The lab started with a bi-specific molecule and then moved to working on a tri-specific one.

Thanks to all the breakthrough laboratories, Sanofi would have one of the most productive scientific teams in pharma. In the years prior to my arrival, to my knowledge, there had been only one paper published in *Science* by any scientist at Sanofi. In the years that followed, we published far more frequently, including the first paper on multifunctional peptides against obesity.

Our trailblazing was encouraged by a CEO, Chris Viehbacher, who believed that novel medicines created strong drug franchises rather than the other way around. Chris and I were in alignment. In my experience, alignment between the CEO and the head of R&D is a key indicator of whether a company will be successful. A company dominated by a CEO who is aligned with their powerful commercial executives is much less likely to succeed.

~

At Sanofi, a predecessor had shut down interactions between the R&D organization and the outside scientific community. Sanofi scientists had been locked in their labs, instructed not to exchange ideas with the outside world. This was a death wish in our field. Great ideas often came from academia and small, leading-edge companies.

As I'd stated publicly, "R&D in pharma has been isolating itself for 20 years, thinking that animal models would be enough and highly predictive, and I think I want to just bring back the discipline of outstanding translational science, which means understand the disease in humans."[3]

We opened the gates and pushed to get fresh ideas and creative individuals into the company. We recruited Andy Plump from Merck, bringing him on as my deputy and senior vice president for research and translational medicine. He would oversee preclinical research. His contributions were invaluable.

A problem we faced was that you couldn't recruit creative workers into a pharma company and keep them creative for long. Soon, they would become bureaucratized and poor at driving innovation. With this reality in mind, in 2013, we established the Sanofi Sunrise initiative to help create and support innovative companies from academia and back early-stage, high-potential science.[4] Katherine Bowdish, Sanofi's vice president of global R&D, led Sunrise. I gave the initiative the name Sunrise because it was supposed to support drug ideas that were rising on the horizon. Our strategy involved taking an equity position in new companies and collaborating with them at arm's length, giving them great autonomy.

At Sanofi, within Sunrise, we had an incentive structure in place that rewarded employee performance and the success of their initiatives (in contrast to the usual, more bureaucratic system common in large pharmaceutical companies). The staff were given more independence. They could scout around the world, looking for opportunities.

Sunrise helped create some exciting new companies. For example, in 2012, with the help of Third Rock Ventures and Greylock Partners,[5] Warp Drive Bio was launched, a "biotechnology company using the molecules and mechanisms of nature to discover and develop transformative medicines."[6] Warp Drive would struggle at first yet ultimately be a success.

Warp Drive Bio was born from the brilliant mind of Harvard chemist Gregory Verdine, who envisioned the assembly (based on gene sequencing) of a large database of natural chemicals with drug potential.[7] To pull off his vision, Verdine had needed funding. On the strong recommendation of Rick Klausner, I'd met Verdine in Paris and personally looked over what he had in mind.[8] He was proposing that many thousands of microbes would have their DNA sequenced, and the information would be compiled into a searchable database, able to aid those hunting for the next potential drug candidate.[9]

Verdine would later recall, "Elias put the Warp Drive project on a rocket sled and shepherded it through Sanofi."[10]

Another company Sanofi-Sunrise helped was MyoKardia, a developer of precision therapies for genetic heart disease.[11] My deputy, Andy Plump, was the one who identified MyoKardia as a great opportunity, and in pursuing it, we again partnered with Third Rock to fund it. In 2014, MyoKardia "entered a worldwide collaboration [with Sanofi] to discover and develop first-of-its-kind targeted therapeutics for heritable heart diseases known as cardiomyopathies, the most common forms of heart muscle disease."[12] Despite MyoKardia's huge potential, I faced criticism from some at Sanofi for supporting the cutting-edge company. Later, following my departure, Sanofi would, unfortunately, move on from MyoKardia. Not long after, Bristol-Myers Squibb would buy MyoKardia for $13.1 billion.[13]

In running R&D, a relatively early challenge I faced was the need to reduce expenses. Patent cliffs and the reality of the current drug portfolio meant a revenue squeeze.[14]

"We'll have to control expenses, which means restructuring every piece of the company, in particular R&D," Chris Viehbacher told me.

Chris wanted my help in trimming R&D. Most of the expense came from employees and research sites. Many of the latter were far too unproductive. We needed to drastically reduce their number.

This wasn't just about cutting costs. It was also about building for to-morrow. Too many of our scientists were not experienced in biologics. To be able to recruit new talent, we had to let go of others. I didn't want any-one to lose their job, yet for Sanofi to survive, we had to move forward.

Although it was headquartered in Paris, Sanofi had become a global company. Our sites in France consumed most of our R&D resources. Yet most of our new drugs were coming from R&D sites in the United States and Germany. We needed to move forward with closing centers in France.

We experienced a huge public backlash. Many of the French unions were horrified by our behavior, which was simply what any CEO in America would do in a heartbeat if they had to save their company. There were demonstrations against us. The protesters hung and burned scare-crows, some with Chris's face on them and others with mine.

The fact that Chris and I were foreigners was not lost on the protes-tors. We faced xenophobic attacks. Chris and I were framed as the killers of French research. It didn't matter that I had convinced Sanofi to invest many billions in French science.

Sanofi's board was pulled into the turmoil, receiving angry calls. In a larger sense, there was a clash between the board and management about what the future of Sanofi looked like. This conflict came to a boil. Eventu-ally, in 2014, Chris was forced to leave.

He was a great CEO. As a leader, he was proactive, had a clear vision and strategy, and took calculated risks. He was an agent of change. The investors believed in him. Sure enough, Sanofi was in far better shape at the end of Chris's tenure than it had been at the start. I knew Chris would be an invaluable addition to whatever organization he went to next.

Not surprisingly, Sanofi's stock collapsed after Chris's exit. Soon, the chair of the board, Serge Weinberg, called and invited me to dinner. I had a good relationship with him and the rest of Sanofi's board. Serge told me that Sanofi wanted to retain me, yet they didn't know who the new CEO would be.

I was approached by some large American companies that wanted me to become their R&D head. They offered much better terms than Sanofi. I turned them down.

My heart was in what we were doing at Sanofi, and I wasn't yet fin-ished. I had recruited some outstanding team members. For me to jump ship would've been unbecoming of a leader. I ultimately agreed to stay on until 2018.

~

With Sanofi in a challenging spot given the crash of its stock and the loss of outside trust in its leadership, Serge asked me to help the company regain its luster.

"Look, the only way I can help is by telling people what we have in the portfolio," I answered. "People are not going to believe speeches. They want to see what drugs we are developing."

I put together an R&D presentation. Meanwhile, it was still unclear who the new CEO would be. Colleagues at Regeneron told me I should apply for the position.

Len Schleifer asserted, "You're making a mistake by not applying. You don't know who they're going to get."

I wasn't sure I wanted to be CEO. It wasn't as interesting as being head of R&D. Also, I wasn't French. The board had decided to bring in a French citizen as the next CEO to reassure the government that Sanofi would stay in France.

While the CEO search continued, I went to Boston and gave my R&D presentation about Sanofi's exciting new portfolio. The presentation worked. Sanofi regained some trust. Things were moving in the right direction.

In 2015, the next CEO was hired. He had plenty of high-level experience in pharma, and although French, he'd spent a large amount of his career in the United States at Pfizer. I hadn't met him before and was unfamiliar with him. Ultimately, our values would not align. I eventually decided that I would finish the important ongoing development programs I conducted and then leave Sanofi by 2018.

~

Although our new CEO did not align with what I felt were the right objectives, R&D managed to succeed. We'd elevated our research expertise, "targeting key therapeutic areas including diabetes, cardiovascular, rare diseases, multiple sclerosis, oncology, immunology and infectious diseases with vaccines."[15] Thirteen new drug approvals had been obtained during my tenure.[16] The R&D organization had transformed into a high-performing one thanks to the efforts of my stellar supporting staff and team.

In 2017, during the Annual Scrip Awards in London, I was awarded the Pharma Executive of the Year Award.[17] I was surprised. To my knowledge, the award wasn't typically given to R&D heads.

It was a testament to the dedication and agility of the extraordinary employees who worked alongside me. I was proud of the work they'd done and would continue to do. The R&D transformation I was being praised for was the sum of many efforts.

~

The board didn't want me to leave Sanofi. Yet I'd made my decision and would stick with it. I'd had a long run at Sanofi and was ready for new challenges. Prior to leaving, I promised to help the CEO find my successor. I had a responsibility to make sure I was replaced by the best possible candidate.

Sanofi had an impressive history. Employees had dedicated their lives to it, many of them colleagues and friends. I didn't want to harm them or the company with my departure.

The CEO and I rigorously searched for the best candidates to replace me. After identifying a small number, I interviewed each one. I told the CEO that I wasn't going to decide on just one person. I was going to give him a choice of two or three candidates who I thought could do the job.

In the end, I proposed two candidates. The CEO decided to go with the exceptional John Reed, whom I knew. I ended my tenure with Sanofi on June 30, 2018.

In 2019, the CEO would leave. Sanofi would change leadership, appointing Paul Hudson the new CEO and marching toward a bright future thanks in part to the successful launch of Dupixent, a biologic we'd developed in close collaboration with Regeneron.

Unretirement and ModeX   23

After stepping down from Sanofi, at 67 years old, I took time to reflect on my past, present, and future. I enjoyed less stress, less travel, and more time with family, including Nadia, children, and grandchildren.

Regarding future work, I'd signed a noncompete agreement with Sanofi that would last several years. Aside from this, I didn't have any limitations on what I could engage in.

I was offered positions on a number of nonprofit boards. I said yes to the Foundation for the NIH and to Research!America, which was still led by the brilliant Mary Woolley. I also joined the board of the Lasker Foundation, a nonprofit whose mission was "to improve health by accelerating support for medical research through recognition of research excellence, advocacy, and education,"[1] utilizing the prestigious Lasker Awards, considered by many to be the equivalent of the Nobel Prize.[2]

During this period, I also engaged in the fight against Alzheimer's. I had a personal connection to the disease, as members of my family had suffered from it, including my late father-in-law. I knew firsthand the devastation it could cause.

Tragically, in the search for a cure, we were failing. George Vradenburg, who I'd known since 2003, was one of the most dedicated and effective advocates for Alzheimer's research. He called me and asked that I share my views on it.

For years, Alzheimer's research had been dominated by the amyloid hypothesis, asserting that a buildup of amyloid β-peptide was the key factor driving pathogenesis.[3] Yet removing the protein hadn't stopped the disease. Moving forward, we needed to examine all areas of possible cause for the disease. We shouldn't leave any stone unturned.

I attended the Lausanne Workshop in 2019, "a highly-curated platform for global Alzheimer's stakeholders to identify challenges, set solution paths, measure progress and hold each other accountable to act."[4] The idea for developing a global mechanism of action against Alzheimer's was raised.[5] I gave a speech, proposing the creation of a global cohort to study the disease in its heterogeneity across the world.

I wanted to vastly increase the number and diversity of patients studied. My observation was that many of the studies, both in the United States and worldwide, were on primarily Caucasian populations. We didn't have a truly global perspective on the disease. Although many were trying to better understand it, most efforts were subscale, subcritical, and overlapping.

As I later told The Hill's Steve Clemons in 2022, "Having 10, 10-foot ladders to try and climb a 100-foot-high wall, will not get you over the wall."[6]

We needed a 100-foot ladder. To obtain it, we needed to come together.

I, along with George Vradenburg, became a founding board member of the Davos Alzheimer's Collaborative, "a global partnership of like-minded organizations that is mobilizing the world against Alzheimer's disease."[7] In "leading the largest global response of its kind," we were "driving progress in three critical areas: developing a global cohort to diversify the populations we can reach with targeted treatments, creating a global clinical trial platform to reduce the cost and time of developing new treatments, and preparing every healthcare system to deliver Alzheimer's care and speed innovations to those who need them most."[8] Despite our best efforts, the world faces a challenging future: "the number of people living with dementia will triple to 139 million (by 2050),"[9] and meanwhile, there will be a dramatic ("up to nine times"[10]) increase in the yearly, $1.3 trillion cost of dementia on the global economy.[11]

As I remained engaged in a variety of new challenges, one of my former colleagues from Sanofi, Gary Nabel, reached out. During my Sanofi tenure, I'd recruited Gary and put him in charge of the Boston breakthrough lab. Unfortunately, Sanofi was going to be cutting costs, to the detriment of the lab. Gary was trying to create a spin-off of it that would exist outside Sanofi. I felt this was a good idea, yet due to the noncompete agreement I'd signed with Sanofi, I couldn't engage in the project at this time.

In the meantime, I was approached by former Sanofi CEO Chris Vieh-bacher, now managing partner of Gurnet Point Capital (GPC), created by Waypoint Capital (which would, in the present, be B-FLEXION), a private, entrepreneurial investment firm founded by Ernesto Bertarelli. Chris asked me to be an adviser for GPC's board, to which I agreed.

Eventually, Ernesto Bertarelli called me with an offer. I'd spent time with him in Geneva and had found him to be exceedingly interesting, intelligent, and brave. I respected his willingness to take risks and tackle huge challenges, his desire to help the planet, and his competitiveness. Regarding the latter, Ernesto, who was an expert sailor, had won the coveted America's Cup in 2003 and 2007.

Over the phone, Ernesto said, "I'd like you to consider joining the management board of Waypoint Capital."

I'd never served as a board member for a capital fund. Finance wasn't my background. Yet Waypoint valued my level of life sciences experience and wanted me to support an effort to drive innovation and advancement in science and medicine.[12] In January 2020, my appointment to Waypoint's board of directors was announced.

I'd never truly seen the world of investments, and it was enjoyable to learn more about it at such a high level. I obtained a more enlightened understanding of the financial world and how it was so important in supporting innovation and the development of new companies. Through working with Waypoint, I gained key knowledge regarding what it took to create an early-stage biotech company, which would prove invaluable in the not-so-distant future.

In March 2020, COVID-19 gripped the world, bringing America into a new, chaotic normal. During the home confinement of the pandemic, I spent time with Nadia and time alone. I reflected on my life. I realized that I yearned to be back in the thick of things. Retirement didn't suit me.

With the pandemic ongoing, I received a call from my former government boss, Alex Azar, who was now the HHS secretary. He'd been talking to Tony Fauci, and they were looking for a way to accelerate the development of a COVID-19 vaccine. The Trump administration was actively searching for someone to take on the role of leading Operation Warp Speed.

I was honored that Azar and Fauci would think of me, yet I was also reluctant to work for the Trump administration as their "therapeutics czar."[13] I did not fully align with the Trump administration's response to the pandemic.[14] Regardless of my feelings, however, leading Operation Warp Speed could be a chance to serve my country in a time of great crisis. I thought I should at least explore the possibility of taking the job.

I met with Azar, Fauci, and Jared Kushner. They were searching for the fastest way to produce a safe, effective vaccine for the American people. The administration wanted it ready before the presidential election in November.[15]

I turned down further consideration for the role for multiple reasons. Although I was willing to do the job for one dollar, costing taxpayers nothing for my services, I felt I wasn't the right fit for it. I had more experience in shaping policy and R&D strategy as opposed to the operational execution of vaccine production. Whoever was hired had to be seasoned in the latter. I thought others, such as the Moroccan immigrant and former head of GSK's vaccine department Moncef Slaoui, had more direct and relevant experience. Slaoui would ultimately be chosen.

Another reason I'd turned down further consideration for the role was that the political pressure associated with the vaccine timetable seemed like trouble, as did the fact that the job of therapeutics czar seemed to lack the authority needed to match its responsibility.

~

As I write this book, the pandemic is over. COVID-19 is taking a back seat to other, more pressing news. It won't, however, be our last pandemic. As I articulated to NPR in 2020 (with some of my wording edited for clarity),

> Pandemic control is going to depend on surveillance of the animal-to-human transfers that we're witnessing around the world. Animal health and human health have to be combined into a surveillance network worldwide, just like you do for weather. We have weather satellites. We have weather stations around the world that exchange data on a harmonized system. That's how you predict hurricanes. . . . The question is, can we do that for global health?[16]

Although this may sound costly to achieve, I can't help but remember an old saying attributed to the philanthropist Mary Lasker: "If you think research is expensive, try disease."[17]

Similarly, to quote Claire Pomeroy from the Lasker Foundation, "If you think preparedness is expensive, try a pandemic."[18]

~

In 2020, with the pandemic ongoing, Gary Nabel and I learned that Sanofi wanted to close the Boston breakthrough lab to save costs. This was a mistake since there was great value in both the lab's technology and the scientists who had developed it.

We pushed for Sanofi to sell the lab rather than shut it down. They tried but couldn't close a deal. By October, Sanofi was ready to shutter the lab. A stellar scientific team was going to be lost—and so much possibility with it. Yet Gary wasn't going to let that happen, and neither was I.

"Let's found a biotech company," I said with conviction.

As a result of my experience in the financial world, I understood how to do this effectively. Gary and I put funding together and cofounded what would be called ModeX Therapeutics, a biotech company that would create cutting-edge, multi-specific biologics. I would be chair of the board, while Gary would be president and CEO. We would be headquartered near Boston.

In assembling ModeX, we hired the team from Sanofi's breakthrough lab, and thanks to the help of Bruce Holbrook, who aided us in swiftly setting up the company in a matter of weeks, we were able to officially open in November. Lab space had been leased, and we brought together all the employees and discussed the future of the company. I told them,

> Sanofi may not be willing to license the technology from the breakthrough lab. So, we must work as if they will not, and come up with our own. . . . The technology you developed at Sanofi is only your phase-one step. You need to invent newer technology capable of more than three specificities. You must go to four, five, or six. The biology we're addressing is complex, and it needs more than one, two, or even three targets to be approached

Within months, our team had formulated a few exceptionally innovative ideas. We patented them. Later, we came to an agreement with Sanofi regarding the use of the technology from the breakthrough lab. This technology was clinically proven. For us, possessing it was an insurance policy.

ModeX was in a stronger position, bolstered by a founding team that included the brilliant Elizabeth Nabel, former director of the National Heart, Lung, and Blood Institute, as well as Zhi-yong Yang, Ronnie Wei, and Chih-Jen Wei, who'd all played key roles in Sanofi's breakthrough lab. John Mascola, then leader of the Vaccine Research Center at the NIH; Ji Zhang, my former COO at Sanofi; and Vijay Chhajlani, an accomplished scientist and pharma leader, were recruited. Our employees were excited, and we gave them the opportunity to buy stock in ModeX. Like a jockey betting on their own horse, our scientists were happy to put their money down on what they believed would be a winner.

Yet due to the rapid progress of our scientific programs, we arrived at an expensive stage of drug development and needed more funding. To complicate matters, the biotech market crashed. These were stormy times for a young biotech company looking for cash.

We felt the best way to move forward was to approach other companies that could be interested in our technology and ask them to partner with us. In January, Gary and I contacted all the R&D heads we knew in the industry. Most immediately responded, wanting to talk. Overall, we were starting 2022 with some momentum. Discussions ensued, and two of the companies were immediately interested in negotiating with us and finding a partnership.

Meanwhile, our scientists were working hard. We met weekly to see their progress. It was exhilarating. This research would be the foundation of a new generation of life-changing biologics. It was significant that we were addressing infectious disease, which had been neglected by the pharma industry. We were also addressing cancer, where the need was still enormous, and autoimmune diseases.

I was learning the different technologies and the manufacturing in a depth that I hadn't at Sanofi. As head of R&D for such a massive organization, I had delegated much to experts. In a small company like ModeX, it was different, however. One had to be involved on a more micro level in every aspect of drug development. I found it fun. For me, it was a period of revival. I felt like I was back in my early research days at Hopkins.

～

With ModeX looking for a company to partner with, what happened next was unexpected. I received a call from the businessman, physician (trained in part at the NIH), and philanthropist Phil Frost, whom I'd known since the mid-2010s. Now well into his eighties, Phil was as sharp, entrepreneurial, and capable as ever. I enjoyed his directness and candor, and his self-made billionaire story was easy to admire. Phil was chair and CEO of the multinational biopharmaceutical and diagnostics company OPKO Health.

Over the phone, Phil said to me, "I need advice for two of my projects. I wonder if you'd be willing to be an adviser or even a board member at OPKO? We need input from someone like you, who has a lot of experience."

"I'm busy with my own company, but I'd be happy to advise you on your projects."

Phil sent me them. I examined them, noting that one was a vaccine project. Gary, a former director of the Vaccine Research Center at NIH, was an expert.

Gary and I visited Phil in Miami to discuss the projects. We went there with absolutely no inkling that ModeX and OPKO might one day come together. Our minds were on Phil's projects. We had a productive meeting.

As part of further evaluating the projects, I called employees working on them. Afterward, I spoke with Phil. During our conversation, Phil inquired about ModeX. I explained more about the company. Interested, Phil requested a confidential deck. He reviewed it.

"Elias, would you mind if I involve some of my board members and advisers in reviewing your company?"

Phil had a Nobel laureate examine ModeX in addition to other top-notch scientific minds. Again, our company impressed.

"Would you do a presentation to the management here?" Phil asked.

In March, Gary and I went down to Miami with our team and presented to OPKO. It went well. In time, after having visited our lab, Phil met with Gary and me. He was willing to acquire ModeX, making the company an independent subsidiary of OPKO and funding it for the next few years.

It was fantastic news, and the transaction made sense. With the acquisition, Phil would significantly upgrade his R&D organization, and we would get funding and the ability to pursue our dreams. On May 9, 2022, it was announced that OPKO had acquired ModeX.

Phil Frost announced, "The acquisition of ModeX Therapeutics significantly broadens our technology foundation and expands our product pipeline to include multi-specific multi-functional antibodies focused on a range of cancers and infectious diseases, with applicability to other therapeutic areas."[19]

COVID-19 and HIV were lead targets, and we were developing a vaccine for Epstein-Barr virus (EBV), which could be the first effective vaccine for this common infectious disease.[20] EBV could cause mononucleosis and was associated with the development of certain cancers and autoimmune diseases.

~

I was now vice chair of the board of directors and president of OPKO. I was back in the command room of a major company, with challenges ahead. It was thrilling. We'd persevere, and in the spring of 2023, OPKO's ModeX would enter into an exclusive worldwide license and collaboration agreement with the pharma giant Merck to develop our novel, multi-targeting EBV vaccine candidate.[21] Later, the government agency BARDA would fund us to further develop our technologies for viral diseases with pandemic potential, including SARS-CoV2 (which causes COVID-19) and influenza.

~

You are who you are. You can't ignore your fundamental identity, and therefore you shouldn't try to live a life that goes against it. During my brief retirement after Sanofi, I was on the sidelines. Yet it didn't suit me. I had to be back in the thick of things and doing more to help others. So at an age when some might slow down, I sped up and found myself in one of the most exciting stages of my career.

Lessons, Science, Immigration, and America

24

On reaching the end of my memoir, I realize that, as a result of having learned the worlds of radiology, academia, government, and industry, I've become like one of ModeX's multifunctional antibodies.

My life shows that you shouldn't limit yourself to a single vocation. Yet you also can't master a million trades at once. To be truly successful at anything, it takes time. I often mastered different vocations one by one.

While doing so, I pursued a "balanced T" approach. The long vertical bar of the T represents the fact that you must be an expert in what you do. You need to have deep knowledge. The horizontal bar of the T represents the fact that you need to be connected to others. Alone, you often can't achieve much. For example, where would I have been without Nadia and my family?

The horizontal bar of the T also represents the reality that you must understand subject matter in fields beyond your own. You need to learn about aspects of the world that seem unrelated to your vocation. It'll make you better at what you do. If you're a doctor, read a work of fiction. If you're a painter, learn about the world of business.

Multi-specificity is important. The world has changed. Complexity has increased. One must be able to grasp their environment as well as the larger context in which their environment is evolving and the changes that are occurring.

∽

The world is contending with disequilibrium from globalization. Tension exists in our political, social, and cultural environment. Tension exists between large nations, like the United States and China.

Disruption is occurring at multiple levels. It was aggravated by the pandemic, the response to which was not extraordinarily effective. Millions of lives were lost, including those of doctors and nurses. There was an increase in inequity, dysfunction, and uncertainty.

How does one approach our troubled world going forward? Science, the understanding of nature, continuous research, continuous technological development for the good of humanity—it all continues to be so important. We are in a race—a race between the emergence of diseases and the cures to beat them, a race between the rise of environmental challenges such as global warming and the potential solutions to overcome them, a race between the nations that seek the destruction of human liberty and those who fight for peace and justice.

It's a race between good and evil. Yet it isn't all black and white. Like everything in life, it has shades of gray.

One of the dangers I see in the world and in our future is a "Manichean"[1] approach to life, which is to say that there is good and bad and nothing in between. Western society is heavily influenced by this black-and-white thinking, and it can lead to devastating prejudice.

The beginning of evil is when one believes that all individuals in a group are equally guilty or liable for the crime of some in that group. Contrary to what Manichean thinking suggests, no group of people is entirely good or entirely bad just as no person is entirely good or entirely bad.

When one simplifies the world into black and white, they create a caricature of reality. They fail to capture the fundamental rocks that lead to a more complete understanding of nature and society. Manichean thinking is a force that can trap us in ignorance.

∽

Contrary to what the ignorant might assert, I believe every individual is precious and deserving of basic human rights. It doesn't matter if they are a Jew or a Muslim or a Christian, man or woman or nonbinary, black or white, old or young. Having traveled around the world countless times and seen societies where the rights of the individual are beneath those of the state, I have a deep appreciation for the United States, which, for now, has a system of law that puts the individual at the center.

The United States is an extraordinary country. It's a place of possibility. It's a place that encourages out-of-the-box thinking and rewards hard work. The meritocracy of this great country gave me a chance to rise high.

Yet America isn't perfect. It has areas where it needs to be so much better, from problems of racism, violence, and xenophobia to the erosion of its meritocracy. Even still, America has much to offer future immigrants no matter their background.

Every immigrant I know says, "America may have some issues, but I love how accepting of differences its citizens can be and that everyone is given opportunities."

This is the greatness of the United States. As a lesson for readers of this book, I want you to come away with a greater appreciation for this wonderful country. Where else but here could an immigrant rise so high? For any immigrants out there looking to forge a successful life in the United States, I want them to know that it can be done.

However, the United States didn't hand me my success. I had to work hard. I also benefited from having been raised in a strong Algerian family that valued education. Additionally, my wife, Nadia, was an invaluable supporter, raised by parents who were among Algeria's best.

The journey of American immigrants is part of a larger story of migration that has been a constant component in the history of mankind. As an immigrant entering the United States, I brought a diverse perspective and set of experiences with me. I wasn't alone in my diversity. Every American is diverse in their own way, just as every human on Earth is as well. We are all a unique experiment of evolution, shaped by environment, education, and culture, among other things.

Have you ever wondered why we are not just clones of each other? Why do we, as a species, have diversity? It's because it makes us stronger. A diversity of perspectives, skills, and insights is an asset.

Some are born to become geniuses like Einstein and have insight into the nature of the universe. Others are born to become prophets, having insight into the nature of human beings. Then there are artists, destined to be the next Beethoven or Mozart. And the masses whose names we might never know bring diversity that is just as important. A man might be born to become a great father and a reliable husband. A daughter might be born to fight for human rights or become a doctor or lawyer. We are all variants of equal value.

∿

I've often asked myself why I was entrusted with some enormous roles throughout my life. Whether it was leading the NIH or Sanofi's R&D, these were responsibilities that exceeded my expectations. I didn't think I would rise so high, yet I did. But why?

My multicultural background allowed me to understand things in a different way than those around me. I have an array of perspectives combined into one. There is Algerian culture in me, passionate, proud, and loving the sea. There is French culture in me, with all its rationalism and determinism. I'm also an American, with an entrepreneurial, pragmatic approach to life.

When it came to moments where I was being considered as a successor for a major position of authority, whether it be at Hopkins or the NIH or Sanofi, I offered a perspective and approach that was different, and I was selected as a result. The unique perspective I brought to the table was also a result of the fact that I never tried to be anything other than myself.

Encouraging people to be themselves rather than forcing them to fit in is essential in helping them make a contribution to society. If we stifle uniqueness, we bury genius.

∿

Whenever I do something paradigm shifting, I'm met with resistance. Every time I wrote a paper that was groundbreaking, there was opposition. The most significant papers in my career were those that I had the most trouble getting initially published.

Rejection can be a mark of importance. It's something you must be ready to face if you are an explorer in science or any other field. And regardless of the likelihood of initial rejection, you shouldn't be shy about your ideas.

Explorers must be brave. They arrive first. They take a risk and discover new land. Pioneers follow them and establish the map of the land, exploring it further. Pioneers shape the future of the land. Once the land is mapped out, the settlers arrive, and they build civilization. Science and other fields follow this process.

∿

So what is currently happening globally in terms of science and technology? The supremacy of the United States is fading because other nations are rising. We would benefit from observing the practices of these nations, identifying what they are doing that works.

Americans alone don't own the truth. We can't thrive through isolation. We are losing ground, and to maintain our lead, we need to make the right decisions going forward.

Meanwhile, in my observation, on a global level, roughly 98 percent of new science and technology is created by 2 percent of scientists. We need to know who these 2 percent are and how to properly train, retain, and encourage them to produce ideas and breakthroughs that neither I nor anybody else can come up with. We need to push them to arrive at the discoveries that can save humanity. We also need to understand science as a truly collaborative enterprise not just within nations but also among them.

Yet not all nations have equal systems of government or equal systems in place to support science and immigrant scientists. The U.S. system of meritocracy and opportunity for immigrants is extraordinary. We have the unique ability to attract the 2 percent of scientists who will make the groundbreaking discoveries of tomorrow. We can enable them to realize their potential.

Although our supremacy in science and technology has faded to a degree, our future remains bright, but not if we shut our doors to immigration. If you look at life sciences in the United States, many of our best and brightest researchers are foreign-born.

China may be a powerful rival on the rise, yet how can they ever truly defeat us if we keep importing the best talent from around the world, including China? It is through immigration that America draws part of its power.

Regarding immigration, the past 50 years in America and in certain countries throughout the world have seen an enormous cultural and intellectual cross-fertilization. On a global scale, societies have also cross-fertilized, and massive intellectual transfers have been made at the highest level. It's global cross-fertilization.

My life story, though seemingly unusual, is just one example of a major trend in our new era. Look around America and see how many CEOs are foreign-born. From Tesla and SpaceX's Elon Musk to Google's Sundar Pichai to Oracle's Safra Catz.

The top 5 percent of intellectual power around the world has changed. There is much more diverse leadership, whether it be in politics or business. Much of a nation's power is now derived from its ability to assemble a truly international leadership community. The societies that do it best, like the United States, have an advantage.

This cross-fertilization, this essential transfer of knowledge, is threatened in both the United States and abroad by rising nationalist, populist forces. These forces threaten immigration. They also, in certain cases, threaten the quality of education.

~

Strong education is an essential part of building a better future. Science, technology, engineering, and math are essential. We need our next generation to know and appreciate these fields. We shouldn't neglect humanities either. We also shouldn't fall into a system of education that is anything but merit based.

Meanwhile, physical sciences, information sciences, data sciences, biological sciences—all of it must be brought together. Multidisciplinary research needs to become the norm, which means that we must change how we organize research in the United States. The notion that we have an agency for this disease, an agency for that disease, another one for this one, and one for energy and one for physics is not the right way to organize ourselves. Convergence of disciplines is what's driving innovation right now. If we want to lead, we must follow what works.

Also, if we want to lead, we must better serve our own population by acknowledging that much of the burden of disease is connected to social and behavioral sciences. Hard sciences cannot be separated from these. We can't succeed in translating what we've achieved scientifically into something of success without an understanding of the social context of the environment we are trying to help.

For example, resistance to technology that could genetically alter mosquitoes, making them unable to carry the malaria parasite, is socially ingrained in certain groups who fear any alteration to the human genome. Thinking with such absolutes is not rational, and addressing this kind of thought process is an integral part of curing a disease. In a larger sense, there seems to be a broad fear of science and technology. Far too many see science as a problem rather than as a solution.

This thinking is fed in part by conspiracy theorists like those who peddle anti-vaccine lies. These lies can lead to deaths. For example, parents preventing their children from being vaccinated for diseases such as measles or polio will pave the way for deadly outbreaks.

However, as alarming as these parents' actions are, we need to communicate the truth to them with patience. Insulting them won't change their minds. Also, in a larger sense, for those who defend science, there needs to be a willingness to communicate facts rather than vague statements. Your scientific truth is not self-evident to everyone. The arrogance and sense of false superiority of elites, whether in the scientific and medical community or others, is a real danger to society.

~

Returning to the subject of my life journey, I've observed that on the road to success, failure cannot be avoided. I've had many failures. Perhaps my greatest one was not spending my early career involved in more fundamental aspects of research.

For example, I wish I had addressed more fundamental questions than diagnosing cancer noninvasively. I now believe that three-quarters of what I published, even if successful, was of limited impact. I should have focused on higher-impact science, on more rocks rather than pebbles or sand.

While it's true that failure cannot be avoided, it's also true that failure can lead to victory. For example, when GE and Siemens turned down my pulmonary nodule reference phantom, this led to the creation of CIRS in 1982, a company that became one of Norfolk's start-up success stories and would continue to better the lives of countless patients and practitioners into the present, long after I was no longer a part of it.

As a scientist, despite wishing I had done certain things differently, I'm proud of my research from when I was a radiologist and a biomedical engineer. In a larger sense, when looking back on my life overall, I'm proud of specific accomplishments, and it reflects that I was driven by specific objectives. I set specific goals and milestones and achieved them.

This is a key part of being successful. For example, my goal at the NIH wasn't simply to "be a great director." It was to achieve specific objectives that would justly serve the agency and the country long after my tenure.

In describing accomplishments, the importance of working with great people cannot be understated. As mentioned earlier in this chapter, the horizontal bar of the "balanced T" represents the fact that you need to be connected to others.

To add to this, it isn't enough to just be connected to anyone. You need to surround yourself with great people. Throughout my life, I had the privilege of working with some extraordinary colleagues. These exceptional individuals shaped my life.

More important than any colleague or friend, however, was the strength and support of my loving wife, Nadia. I wouldn't have been able to achieve all that I have without her. She was—and is—an essential part of my story, from the days of our courtship in Algiers and into the present.

Nadia has always had a generous heart, and her continued involvement in the Zerhouni Family Charitable Foundation (which we founded in 2002) demonstrates this. Our foundation has given to a number of key organizations, such as the American Civil Liberties Union, the World Wildlife Fund, the FNIH, and the Maryland Food Bank, among others. Nadia is a guiding force in our foundation, and she strongly believes in the importance of giving to others.

Through decades of practicing pediatric endocrinology and balancing the demands of mothering our children, often in my absence, Nadia has given so much to our family, so much of her love, dedication, and guidance. I'm thankful for her and for my children, Will, Yasmin, and Adam, who have, with the help of their steadfast mother, grown to become such wonderful adults.

~

With my memoir reaching its end, I want to leave you with a final lesson: the power of compassion. On that early morning in 1962 in Pointe Pescade, Dr. Kollen knocked on my family's door, warning us we were next on the list of Algerians to be killed. I wonder if he or the Pied Noir taxi driver Mr. Rosello, who warned him, could've imagined the meaning of the lives they were saving. I wonder if my brave uncle, Djillali, who was badly wounded by a French attack in the war, could have known, as he struggled to survive in the desert, the effect his survival and subsequent mentorship would have on my life.

Our actions echo forever, and though our lives are no more than a blink in the history of humanity, no more than a grain of sand in a sweeping Algerian desert, they matter. What we do for others matters.

In recounting my life to you, its trajectory and its highs and lows, I hope the lessons will be helpful in your own journey—the importance of being bold and taking calculated risks; of curiosity and asking questions; of a rock, pebble, sand approach to life; and of "disease knows no politics."

I want you to use these lessons in your own way. It doesn't matter whether you're like me, whether you're a Democrat or a Republican, or whether you're a Muslim or a Jew. I just want all people to live the best life they can to the best of their abilities. I suppose that's the physician in me, looking to help and heal, even long after I've left this Earth.

Epilogue
From Health Care to Hell Care

My life journey took me through multiple components of the U.S. health care system. I observed it through the lens of industry, academia, and government. On my arrival in 1975, I felt America's health care system was the greatest in the world. In the coming decades, I was saddened to witness its transformation from health care to hell care.

How is it that the system evolved to the point of becoming a huge burden to the nation and millions of patients? Opaque, complex, and more expensive than any comparable system in developed nations, the United States now ranks last on many important health indicators. An observation shared with me recently was that during one of the peaks of the Cold War, defense spending climbed to around 9 percent of the nation's gross domestic product (GDP). Today, defense spending is around 3 percent of GDP, whereas as of 2022, health care spending has ballooned to be 17.3 percent of GDP (and rising). This is far more than what other developed nations spend. We pay more and get less.

The worry I hear from policymakers and economists is that servicing our debt and paying for rising health care costs is more threatening to our country's well-being than inflation and insufficient economic productivity. So dysfunctional is our health care system that it is now hurting countless doctors, in addition to patients, burning out the former through arcane complexity. Doctors must obtain burdensome and time-consuming pre-authorizations designed to limit care. The control over the practice of medicine has shifted to obscure management methods in giant, for-profit insurance systems.

These systems leave millions of patients afraid of increasingly frequent coverage denials.

I hear from suffering patients who are striving to avoid any contact with our health care system for fear of surprise bills and being chased by debt collectors capable of taking them to court and ruining their lives. Yet skipping preventive care merely punts problems down the road, leaving both the insured and the millions of uninsured to crowd expensive emergency rooms for conditions that could have been averted.

Even if a patient is willing and able to pay the exorbitant prices of this system, there is no guarantee they can find a doctor. We are in short supply of physicians, including those in primary care. I've experienced this problem firsthand. After my longtime Hopkins primary care physician retired, I could not easily find a replacement. I'm a former NIH director, with vast connections in the world of medicine, and even still, it wasn't easy.

During my NIH tenure, the issue of helping seniors receive Medicare coverage for prescription drugs was front and center in the White House and Congress. Some seniors were choosing between buying food or their medicine. It was a demeaning dilemma for America's greatest generation. They'd stormed the beaches of Normandy only to starve so they could afford their pills.

All parties agreed that having seniors go hungry to pay for medicines was unbecoming of our great nation. Yet in the ensuing political battles, extension of this basic Medicare benefit narrowly passed through Congress. Here, partisanship and politics and special interests had infected themselves into the treatment of disease.

Likewise, following my NIH tenure, I witnessed the heated battles around Obamacare with dismay. Extending coverage to more Americans should have been a no-brainer, yet here again, the legislation narrowly passed in Congress (and continues to be viciously attacked). If popular additional basic benefits like drug coverage for seniors or insurance coverage for millions of Americans struggled to get through Congress, then what would happen if a larger reform of health care involved any restrictions of benefits? How could any congressman, congresswoman, or president willing to tackle this grave issue and face dire political retributions succeed?

During my NIH tenure, I remember visiting Mitch Daniels, director of the Office of Management and Budget (who would go on to become governor of Indiana). Mitch had a painting in his office of a child climbing on a runaway train to try to stop it.

"The train will crash if the child can't get to the brakes soon," Mitch stated.

In his metaphor, the runaway train was the national budget and grow-ing deficits, and Mitch was the child trying to stop the coming wreck. It was his way of arguing for reducing the NIH budget, which I vehemently opposed. Regardless, the metaphor stuck with me.

Any politician trying to solve the health care crisis can't help but seem like a child on a runaway train. And despite the runaway spending on health care, this country still does not deliver satisfactory services, particu-larly to poor or underserved populations.

Why is this? What could be a solution? Is there a solution? I've at-tended dozens of meetings and discussions with HHS, White House, and congressional officials as well as health care think tanks and economists. I've attended conferences, read publications by experienced authors, and heard pundits and companies propose solutions, all of which promised better results yet have not delivered. Despite changes, our crisis rages on.

$\sim$

Drug prices are one piece of the problem. During my tenure at Sanofi, I saw firsthand how drug prices varied across the world, with U.S. patients regularly paying much more for branded drugs than citizens of other countries. This cost burden pushed some U.S. patients to try to reimport medicines (created in majority by the U.S. R&D ecosystem) from coun-tries where prices were much lower.

"Why do we charge more in the United States?" I asked Sanofi colleagues.

I was told by the then CEO of Sanofi, Chris Viehbacher, that in the United States, if Sanofi charged $100 for a drug, they collected only $45, as there were so many intermediaries, such as insurance companies, phar-macy benefit managers, and others, that extracted a premium from the sale of Sanofi's products. Meanwhile, in Europe, if Sanofi charged $100, they collected $90.

As for the powerful intermediaries extracting value in the United States, these bad actors threatened to not cover the drugs of pharma companies that tried to reduce their prices (as it would cut into the intermediaries' revenues). The U.S. system had become concentrated into the hands of a small number of gigantic health insurance companies and pharmacy benefit managers, forming monopolies that even giant pharmaceutical companies or providers had little power against.

When it came to the cost of drugs, I was curious why prices for exist-ing ones were regularly raised far above the costs of inflation in the United States by pharmaceutical companies. Sometimes this would happen twice in a year in the absence of any significant innovation to the drug being sold. The price increases, I was told, were to make sure that pharma companies could fund the rising costs of R&D and satisfy the intermediaries for whom higher prices provided more revenues.

This was a stunning discovery for me. I understood the reasoning, however selfish, of each of the decisions made by each actor in the system. Yet in the end, who really paid? American patients. And who was our health care system really caring for? Corporations. This was insane. I observed that the sum of rational decisions by rational actors could lead to irrational outcomes.

Drug prices aren't the only inflated expense that U.S. patients must endure. The cost of care is also on a runaway train, having reached staggering heights.

During my tenure with Sanofi, I spent significant time in France, allowing me to compare health care there with what we had in America. In France, my best friend from high school developed pancreatic cancer and was operated on, treated, and survived for five years. I asked him what his total out-of-pocket expense was. It was less than €10,000. I was shocked. The same treatment might cost hundreds of thousands of dollars in the United States.

Ambulatory expenses were no exception to the price disparity. In the United States, the price of an ambulance could be 30 times greater than it was in France. My own mother had a heart attack in Paris, was transported by ambulance to a nearby hospital, and was treated within three hours with a rapid catheter intervention that saved her heart. The total cost she paid was less than €500.

When comparing the United States and other developed countries, the price disparity for routine procedures is colossal. Why? In the United States, a lack of pricing transparency, costly provider bureaucracies, and hospital monopolies all feed the problem. Yet well-intentioned legislation also contributes.

For example, early in my career, I participated in lobbying Congress to limit the performance of mammography to certified radiologists with special training in mammography. The intention was good and rational: protecting the public from poor-quality tests. Congress agreed and passed the legislation. Unfortunately, our rational choices would yield an irrational outcome. The legislation unintentionally led to a professional monopoly on mammography, limiting the procedure to a small number of providers and leading to an increase in costs and reduced access.

In another example of legislation gone awry, rational and well-intentioned lobbying by gastroenterologists convinced Congress to limit the performance of colonoscopies to only specially trained gastroenterologists. At the time, the procedure had a high risk of perforation to the colon. The legislation was rational, yet it led to a provider monopoly that would make colonoscopies cost over 10 times more than they did in other developed countries, even as the procedure became safer and easier to administer.

In contrast to the United States, in Japan, for example, a single doctor can supervise several specially trained assistants via real-time video as they perform colonoscopies. The supervising gastroenterologist intervenes only when a lesion needs to be resected, which costs a patient only a few hundred dollars. Meanwhile, in the United States, a routine colonoscopy can cost more than $4,000.

～

Again and again, in the United States, rational legislative decisions that are centrally imposed on the entire country lead to irrational and costly consequences. Clearly, lobbying Congress to be granted special regulations can create monopolies on certain care, disturbing the balance between demand and supply and stifling the innovation needed to better serve patients.

In addition, the failure of the federal government to maintain competition in health care, via the antitrust powers of the Federal Trade Commission, has led to giant monopolies that wield immense influence over politicians and the executive and legislative branches of our government. In some cities, large hospital corporations formed by mergers (an initially rational decision) to resist the oligopolistic power of insurance companies have irrationally driven up costs for all Americans. Disturbingly, the compensation of executives in some of these allegedly nonprofit health systems rivals that of CEOs in for-profit corporations.

I can't help but conclude that the fundamental reason no one and no government has been able to tame this runaway health care system is that well-intentioned congressional and government regulations (or lack thereof) have had the consequence of making the system captive to powerful vested interests. These vested interests, acting in rational self-interest, prevent meaningful reform of our irrational system.

～

Among its many flaws, our irrational system fails to meet the varying needs of patients. As I visited many parts of the country as NIH director, it became apparent to me that the health care needs of different regions were radically different. For example, the epidemiology of regions like the Mississippi delta contrasted immensely with those of Colorado or Minnesota. In the end, I was puzzled as to why anyone would think a one-size-fits-all health care system shaped by policymakers in Washington could effectively address the contrasting regional, epidemiological differences of our country.

As a physician, I believe that solutions should be tailored to the reality of a disease in the relevant population. Our country is too heterogeneous and too large to believe that the same policies will be equally effective across every region. Countries with smaller populations, such as the United Kingdom, Germany, and Canada, manage their health care regionally, with a base of central regulatory policies but no overbearing central micromanagement.

As a physician, I also believe that patients are served best when they are heard. Right now, they aren't. Whenever I've attended meetings regarding health care, I'm struck by the absence, at the table, of the supposed ultimate beneficiaries of our system: patients. The adage "if you are not at the table, you'll be on the menu" comes to mind. It is patients who are on the menu of a gluttonous health care system.

~

The thoughts I've expressed in this chapter are ones I've kept in the dark for too long, spoken only to colleagues. I've hesitated to publicly express them, as I know I'll be attacked for it. I also couldn't come up with a solution for the crisis. I kept hoping that the real experts, whom I knew to be extremely competent, would eventually get it right. But that has not happened.

So can our system be progressively changed? I've come to the conclusion that the system is designed to give us the results we observe and will be hard to change without a fundamental redesign.

After reflecting about what the real "rocks" are to achieve positive change, I concluded that the following four would be central:

1. Find a way to depoliticize health care.
2. Decentralize health care to fit the needs of the different regions of the country.
3. Disintermediate the system to reduce non–value-added costs.
4. Encourage and protect innovation in health care delivery.

Easier said than done. Experts might call my thinking wishful and naïve. They might say these goals are impossible in our highly partisan political system. They are wrong. We can succeed, though it will not be easy.

Earlier in its history, the United States performed an unthinkable, seemingly "impossible" system transformation. The Federal Reserve System, established in 1913, with its 12 regional banks, serves the differing needs of different areas of the country while retaining common parameters for all. The Federal Reserve enjoys autonomy and distance from political pressures that might hinder its effectiveness and pollute its objectives.

The idea I would like to propose here is to restructure our health care system along the design of the Federal Reserve. Actually, this idea is not new. I am told that some legislators did suggest such an approach in the past. More recently, Bill Brody told me that he had suggested a similar approach at the time of the Obamacare reforms in 2010.

The central idea is that we need not a revolution but instead a devolution of our captive health care system back to the people. Essentially, Congress would create and appoint a national health care governor, operating with political independence to set federal policy in cooperation with 10 to 12 regional health care governors, having their own authority to adapt the health care system of their region to address the specific needs of their population.

These regions should comprise a sufficient number of patients in order to enable proper insurance mechanisms while not being so large as to make effective management impossible. Each region should have a governing health care advisory board that includes patient representatives. Finally, the patient would have a seat at the table rather than being on the menu.

Key to this new system is a basic package of health care services, with affordable co-pay levels, that should be available to all citizens regardless of income, employment status, age, or any other consideration. The delivery of services, inherent to this basic health care package, should be managed by each regional governor and funded mostly by the federal government. Additional public or private insurance can be developed and provided to supplement the basic federal package.

Each region should be free to allow innovative health care approaches to be tested and implemented in their system. By devolving health care away from a centralized approach, I'm sure that multiple approaches and innovations will be tested and the best ones adopted around the country rather than being stifled by heavy and uniform regulations.

Obviously, when it comes to this reform, the devil will be in the details. And as always, I am a realist. The chances of such a reform being passed and enacted are very slim, but why not? What is the worst that can happen?

In the end, however, without a grassroots, take-it-to-the-streets movement by the citizens of this country to get our political leaders to address
this crisis, change will not happen. And without strong leadership by a
president and Congress focused on the four "rocks of change" (depoliti-
cization, decentralization [regionalization], disintermediation, and genuine
American innovation), the runaway train of health care is unlikely to get
back on track.

Notes

Foreword

1. Elias Zerhouni, "The NIH Roadmap," *Science* 302, no. 5642 (2003): 63–72, https://doi.org/10.1126/science.1091867.

2. Elias Zerhouni, "The NIH Reform Act of 2006: Progress, Challenges, and Next Steps," news releases, NIH, September 9, 2008, https://www.nih.gov/news-events/news-releases/nih-reform-act-2006-progress-challenges-next-steps.

3. I. J. Good, *The Scientist Speculates* (New York: Basic Books, 1962).

Introduction

1. "NIH Director Nomination," C-Span, April 30, 2002, https://www.c-span.org/video/?169822-1/nih-director-nomination.

Chapter 1. Childhood and the War

1. Michael Kimmelman, "Footprints of Pieds-Noirs Reach Deep into France," *New York Times*, March 5, 2009, https://www.nytimes.com/2009/03/05/world/europe/05iht-kimmel.4.20622745.html.

2. Alistair Horne, *A Savage War of Peace: Algeria 1954–1962* (New York: New York Review Books, 2011), 492, Kindle.

3. Horne, *A Savage War of Peace*, Battle of Algiers, Kindle.

4. "Algerian War: Macron in Rare Torture Admission," BBC, September 13, 2018, https://www.bbc.com/news/world-europe-45513842.

5. James McDougall, *A History of Algeria* (Cambridge: Cambridge University Press, 2017), 144, Kindle.

6. McDougall, *A History of Algeria*, 226, Kindle.

Chapter 2. The Blue Night

1. James McDougall, *A History of Algeria* (Cambridge: Cambridge University Press, 2017), 227, Kindle.

Chapter 3. Independence and Teenage Years

1. James McDougall, *A History of Algeria* (Cambridge: Cambridge University Press, 2017), Pouvoir, Putsch, and the Charismatic State, Kindle.

2. McDougall, *A History of Algeria*, Pouvoir, Putsch, and the Charismatic State, Kindle.

Chapter 4. The University of Algiers

1. James McDougall, *A History of Algeria* (Cambridge: Cambridge University Press, 2017), 251, Kindle.

Chapter 5. Radiology, Love, and Loss

1. Edmund S. Higgins, "Fifty Years Ago, the First CT Scan Let Doctors See Inside a Living Skull," *Smithsonian Magazine*, October 1, 2021, https://www.smithsonianmag.com/innovation/fifty-years-ago-the-first-ct-scan-let-doctors-see-inside-a-living-skull-180978792.

2. "History," Educational Commission for Foreign Medical Graduates, last updated February 10, 2023, https://www.ecfmg.org/about/history.html.

Chapter 6. Johns Hopkins Radiology

1. Andrew H. Beck, "The Flexner Report and the Standardization of American Medical Education," *JAMA* 291, no. 17 (2004): 2139–40, https://doi.org/10.1001/jama.291.17.2139.

2. Thomas P. Duffy, "The Flexner Report—100 Years Later," *Yale Journal of Biology and Medicine* 84, no. 3 (2011): 269–76, https://www.ncbi.nlm.nih.gov/pmc/articles/PMC3178858.

3. Duffy, "The Flexner Report."

4. "'Father of Modern Medicine': The Johns Hopkins School of Medicine, 1889–1905," National Library of Medicine Profiles in Science, NIH, accessed August 28, 2023, https://profiles.nlm.nih.gov/spotlight/gf/feature/father-of-modern-medicine-the-johns-hopkins-school-of-medicine-1889-1905.

Chapter 7. Residency and a Dying Algerian President

1. "Elias A. Zerhouni, MD, Radiologist: New Director of the National Institutes of Health," *Radiology* 224, no. 2 (2002): 309, https://doi.org/10.1148/radiol.2242020547.

Chapter 8. Eastern Virginia Medical School and Becoming an Entrepreneur and Inventor

1. To succinctly quote the National Institute of Standards and Technology, "In the biomedical research community, medical imaging phantoms are objects used as stand-ins for human tissues to ensure that systems and methods for imaging the human body are operating correctly." For more information, see "What Are Imaging Phantoms?," National Institute of Standards and Technology, updated January 24, 2024, https://www.nist.gov/physics/what-are-imaging-phantoms.

2. E. A. Zerhouni, F. P. Stitik, S. S. Siegelman, D. P. Naidich, S. S. Sagel, A. V. Proto, J. R. Muhm, J. W. Walsh, C. R. Martinez, and R. T. Heelan, "CT of the Pulmonary Nodule: A Cooperative Study," *Radiology* 160, no. 2 (August 1, 1986): 319–27, https://doi.org/10.1148/radiology.160.2.3726107.

3. Zerhouni et al., "CT of the Pulmonary Nodule."

Chapter 9. A CT Microscope

1. Ryan Bradley, "This Is Your Brain on . . . Surgical Sound Waves," *Fortune*, June 12, 2014, https://fortune.com/2014/06/12/focused-ultrasound-surgery.

2. "E. Robert Heitzman, MD, Former RSNA President, Dies at 93," RSNA News, Radiological Society of North America, November 12, 2020, https://www.rsna.org/news/2020/october/in-memoriam-robert-heitzman#.

3. UPI, "Andres Gruentzig Dies in Air Crash," *New York Times*, October 29, 1985, https://www.nytimes.com/1985/10/29/us/andres-gruentzig-dies-in-air-crash.html.

Chapter 12. The Challenges of Managed Care and Becoming a National Cancer Institute Adviser

1. Ed Miller, interview, July 19, 2024.

2. M. William Salganik, "JH Medical Selects Chief Financial Officer Grossi Is Promoted by Entity Now Overseeing Med School, Health System," *Baltimore Sun*, August 31, 2023, https://www.baltimoresun.com/news/bs-xpm-1996-09-21-1996265088-story.html.

Chapter 13. Pulse Management

1. "Our Commitment," Abell Foundation, accessed August 5, 2024, https://abell.org.

2. Sarah Koenig and David Nitkin, "Howard 'Pete' Rawlings Dies at 66," *Baltimore Sun*, November 14, 2003, https://msa.maryland.gov/megafile/msa/speccol/sc3500/sc3520/012200/012298/html/sun14nov2003.html.

3. Greg Rienzi, "Biotech Park to Rise in East Baltimore," *Gazette*, April 22, 2002, https://pages.jh.edu/gazette/2002/22apr02/22biotec.html.

4. Rienzi, "Biotech Park to Rise in East Baltimore."

5. Rienzi, "Biotech Park to Rise in East Baltimore."

Chapter 14. The White House Is on the Line

1. "Who We Are," NIH, accessed August 1, 2024, https://www.nih.gov/about-nih/who-we-are.

2. Research!America, accessed August 27, 2023, https://www.research america.org/who-we-are.

3. "President Nominates NIH Director and Surgeon General," Office of the Press Secretary, White House Archives of President George W. Bush, March 26, 2002, https://georgewbush-whitehouse.archives.gov/news/releases/2002/03/20020326-3.html.

4. "President Nominates NIH Director and Surgeon General."

5. "President Nominates NIH Director and Surgeon General."

6. "President Nominates NIH Director and Surgeon General."

7. "Surgeon General Nomination," C-Span, March 26, 2002, https://www.c-span.org/video/?169340-1/surgeon-general-nomination.

Chapter 15. Confirmation

1. "NIH Director Nomination," C-Span, April 30, 2002, https://www.c-span.org/video/?169822-1/nih-director-nomination.

2. "NIH Director Nomination."

3. "NIH Director Nomination."

4. "NIH Director Nomination."

5. "NIH Director Nomination."

6. "NIH Director Nomination."

7. "NIH Director Nomination."

8. "NIH Director Nomination."

9. "NIH Director Nomination."

10. "NIH Director Nomination."

11. "NIH Director Nomination."

12. "NIH Director Nomination."

13. "NIH Director Nomination."

14. "NIH Director Nomination."

15. "NIH Director Nomination."

16. "NIH Director Nomination."

17. "NIH Director Nomination."

18. "NIH Director Nomination."

19. "NIH Director Nomination."

20. "NIH Director Nomination."

21. "NIH Director Nomination."

22. "NIH Director Nomination."

23. "NIH Director Nomination."

24. "NIH Director Nomination."

25. "NIH Director Nomination."

26. "NIH Director Nomination."

27. "NIH Director Nomination."
28. "NIH Director Nomination."
29. "NIH Director Nomination."
30. "NIH Director Nomination."
31. "NIH Director Nomination."
32. "NIH Director Nomination."
33. "NIH Director Nomination."
34. "NIH Director Nomination."
35. "NIH Director Nomination."
36. "NIH Director Nomination."
37. "NIH Director Nomination."
38. "NIH Director Nomination."
39. "NIH Director Nomination."
40. "NIH Director Nomination."
41. "NIH Director Nomination."
42. "NIH Director Nomination."
43. "NIH Director Nomination."
44. "NIH Director Nomination."
45. "NIH Director Nomination."
46. "NIH Director Nomination."
47. "NIH Director Nomination."
48. "NIH Director Nomination."
49. "NIH Director Nomination."
50. "NIH Director Nomination."
51. "NIH Director Nomination."

Chapter 16. Building a Roadmap for Twenty-First-Century Medical Research

1. Denise Grady, "A Conversation with: Elias Zerhouni; Learning the Science of Leading," *New York Times,* July 15, 2003, https://www.nytimes.com/2003/07/15/science/a-conversation-with-elias-zerhouni-learning-the-science-of-leading.html.
2. Grady, "A Conversation with: Elias Zerhouni."
3. William Brody, interviewed by Edward Kriz, November, 4, 2022.
4. Elias Zerhouni, "The NIH Roadmap," *Science* 302, no. 5642 (2003): 63–72, https://doi.org/10.1126/science.1091867.
5. Zerhouni, "The NIH Roadmap."
6. Zerhouni, "The NIH Roadmap."
7. Zerhouni, "The NIH Roadmap."
8. Zerhouni, "The NIH Roadmap."
9. Zerhouni, "The NIH Roadmap."
10. Zerhouni, "The NIH Roadmap."
11. Zerhouni, "The NIH Roadmap."
12. Zerhouni, "The NIH Roadmap."

13. Zerhouni, "The NIH Roadmap."

14. Elias Zerhouni, "The NIH Reform Act of 2006: Progress, Challenges, and Next Steps," news releases, NIH, September 9, 2008, https://www.nih.gov /news events/news-releases/nih-reform-act-2006-progress-challenges-next-steps.

15. Zerhouni, "The NIH Roadmap."

16. Zerhouni, "The NIH Roadmap."

17. Zerhouni, "The NIH Roadmap."

18. Zerhouni, "The NIH Roadmap."

19. Zerhouni, "The NIH Roadmap."

20. Meredith Wadman, "Early Success Claimed for Zerhouni's NIH Roadmap," *Nature* 431, no. 886 (2004), https://doi.org/10.1038/431886b.

Chapter 17. The Gates Foundation, Congress, and the U.S. President's Emergency Plan for AIDS Relief

1. "About Grand Challenges Initiatives," Grand Challenges, accessed August 17, 2023, https://www.grandchallenges.org/about.

2. H. Varmus, R. Klausner, E. Zerhouni, T. Acharya, A. S. Daar, and P. A. Singer, "Grand Challenges in Global Health," *Science* 302, no. 5644 (2003): 398–99, https://doi.org/10.1126/science.1091769.

3. "Fourteen Grand Challenges in Global Health Announced in $200 Million Initiative," Bill & Melinda Gates Foundation, accessed August 17, 2023, https:// www.gatesfoundation.org/Ideas/Media-Center/Press-Releases/2003/10/14 -Grand-Challenges-in-Global-Health.

4. Varmus et al., "Grand Challenges in Global Health."

5. "About Grand Challenges Initiatives."

6. Anthony S. Fauci, MD, and Robert W. Eisinger, PhD, "PEPFAR—15 Years and Counting the Lives Saved," *New England Journal of Medicine* 378 (2018): 314–16, https://doi.org/10.1056/NEJMp1714773.

7. Peter Wehner, "My Friend, Mike Gerson," *The Atlantic*, November 18, 2022, https://www.theatlantic.com/ideas/archive/2022/11/michael-gerson -speechwriter-george-bush-dies-cancer/672172.

8. Fauci and Eisinger, "PEPFAR."

9. Fauci and Eisinger, "PEPFAR."

10. Compiled by the Office of NIH History, Office of Communications and Public Liaison, and Office of the Director, *NIH Events 2003–2004, Elias A. Zerhouni, MD, Director* (2003–2004).

11. Crystal Cazier and Andrew Kaufmann, "An Oral History of PEPFAR: How a 'Dream Big' Partnership Is Saving the Lives of Millions," Goerge W. Bush Presidential Center, February 24, 2023, https://www.bushcenter.org/pub lications/an-oral-history-of-pepfar-how-a-dream-big-partnership-is-saving-the -lives-of-millions.

Chapter 18. Bioterrorism, Pandemic Threats, and a Conflict-of-Interest Crisis

1. "Amerithrax or Anthrax Investigation," History, FBI, accessed August 17, 2023, http://www.fbi.gov/history/famous-cases/amerithrax-or-anthrax-investigation.

2. "S.3678—Pandemic and All-Hazards Preparedness Act," 109th Congress (2005–2006), Congress.gov, accessed August 17, 2023, https://www.congress.gov/bill/109th-congress/senate-bill/3678.

3. "Pandemic and All Hazards Preparedness Act (PAHPA)," Administration for Strategic Preparedness and Response, HHS.gov, accessed August 17, 2023, https://www.phe.gov/preparedness/legal/pahpa/pages/default.aspx.

4. Compiled by the Office of NIH History, Office of Communications and Public Liaison, and Office of the Director, *NIH Events 2004–2005, Elias A. Zerhouni, MD, Director* (2004–2005).

5. David Willman, "Stealth Merger: Drug Companies and Government Medical Research," *Los Angeles Times*, December 7, 2003, https://www.latimes.com/archives/la-xpm-2003-dec-07-na-nih7-story.html.

6. Willman, "Stealth Merger."

7. Jonathan Knight, "Accusations of Bias Prompt NIH Review of Ethical Guidelines," *Nature* 426, no. 741 (2003), https://doi.org/10.1038/426741a.

8. Knight, "Accusations of Bias Prompt NIH Review of Ethical Guidelines."

9. Erika Check, "Ethics Accusations Spark Rapid Reaction from NIH Chief," *Nature* 427, no. 187 (2004), https://doi.org/10.1038/427187b.

10. Check, "Ethics Accusations Spark Rapid Reaction from NIH Chief."

11. Robert Steinbrook, MD, "Financial Conflicts of Interest and the NIH," *New England Journal of Medicine* 350 (2004): 327–30, https://doi.org/10.1056/NEJMp038247.

12. David Willman and Jon Marino, "NIH Directors No Longer Drug Firm Consultants," *Los Angeles Times*, January 23, 2004, https://www.latimes.com/archives/la-xpm-2004-jan-23-na-nih23-story.html.

13. Compiled by the Office of NIH History, Office of Communications and Public Liaison, and Office of the Director, *NIH Events 2003–2004, Elias A. Zerhouni, MD, Director* (2003–2004).

14. William Brody, interviewed by Edward Kriz, November 4, 2022.

15. Compiled by the Office of NIH History.

16. Compiled by the Office of NIH History.

17. Compiled by the Office of NIH History.

18. William Brody, interviewed by Edward Kriz.

19. *NIH Ethics Concerns: Consulting Arrangements and Outside Awards: Hearings before the Subcommittee on Oversight and Investigations of the Committee on Energy and Commerce House of Representatives, One Hundred Eighth Congress, Second Session, May 12, May 18, and June 22, 2004* (Washington, DC: U.S. Government Printing Office, 2004), 3–5.

20. *NIH Ethics Concerns*, 6.
21. *NIH Ethics Concerns*, 8.
22. *NIH Ethics Concerns*, 12.
23. Compiled by the Office of NIH History.
24. Former NIH legislative aide Marc Smolonsky, e-mail to the author/comments on the manuscript, July 18, 2023.
25. Former NIH legislative aide Marc Smolonsky.
26. Former NIH legislative aide Marc Smolonsky.
27. "Sunshine Act," Johns Hopkins University & Medicine, last updated November 2022, https://industryinteraction.jhu.edu/sunshine-act.

Chapter 19. Pioneers and Political Interference

1. Jeremy Berg, notes to the author, July 22, 2024.
2. Jeremy Berg, notes to the author, July 22, 2024.
3. "NIH Director's Pioneer Award Recipients, 2005 Awardees," NIH Director's Pioneer Award, NIH, last reviewed on July 23, 2021, https://commonfund.nih.gov/pioneer/AwardRecipients05.
4. "NIH Director's Pioneer Award Recipients, 2005 Awardees."
5. Michael Häusser, "Optogenetics—The Might of Light," *New England Journal of Medicine* 385 (2021): 1623–26, https://doi.org/10.1056/NEJMcibr2111915.
6. Jeremy Berg, notes to the author, July 22, 2024.
7. Former NIH legislative aide Marc Smolonsky, e-mail to the author/comments on the manuscript, July 18, 2023.
8. Former NIH legislative aide Marc Smolonsky.
9. Former NIH legislative aide Marc Smolonsky.
10. Matt Schudel, "Louis P. Sheldon, Inflammatory Anti-Gay Crusader of 'Traditional Values,' Dies at 85," *Washington Post*, June 6, 2020, https://www.washingtonpost.com/local/obituaries/louis-p-sheldon-inflammatory-anti-gay-crusader-of-traditional-values-dies-at-85/2020/06/06/20fcb81a-a80d-11ea-bb20-ebf0921f3bbd_story.html.
11. Jocelyn Kaiser, "NIH Roiled by Inquiries over Grants Hit List," *Science* 302, no. 5646: 758 (2003), https://doi.org/10.1126/science.302.5646.758.
12. Kaiser, "NIH Roiled by Inquiries over Grants Hit List."
13. Kaiser, "NIH Roiled by Inquiries over Grants Hit List."
14. Kaiser, "NIH Roiled by Inquiries over Grants Hit List."
15. Kaiser, "NIH Roiled by Inquiries over Grants Hit List."
16. Jocelyn Kaiser, "Sex Studies 'Properly' Approved," *Science* 303, no. 5659 (2004): 741, https://doi.org/10.1126/science.303.5659.741a.
17. Kaiser, "Sex Studies 'Properly' Approved."
18. Kaiser, "Sex Studies 'Properly' Approved."
19. Compiled by the Office of NIH History, Office of Communications and Public Liaison, and Office of the Director, *NIH Events 2003–2004, Elias A. Zerhouni, MD, Director* (2003–2004).

20. Fiona Ortiz and Justin Madden, "Ex-House Speaker Hastert Gets 15 Months, Admits Sex Abuse," Reuters, April 27, 2016, https://www.reuters.com/article/us-crime-hastert-idUSKCN0XO178.

21. Former NIH legislative aide Marc Smolonsky.

22. Former NIH legislative aide Marc Smolonsky.

Chapter 20. The Reform Act, Stem Cells, the French, and Cruising to the Finish Line

1. Elias Zerhouni, "The NIH Reform Act of 2006: Progress, Challenges, and Next Steps," news releases, NIH, September 9, 2008, https://www.nih.gov/news-events/news-releases/nih-reform-act-2006-progress-challenges-next-steps.

2. Zerhouni, "The NIH Reform Act of 2006."

3. Former NIH legislative aide Marc Smolonsky, e-mail to the author/comments on the manuscript, July 18, 2023.

4. Former NIH legislative aide Marc Smolonsky.

5. Former NIH legislative aide Marc Smolonsky.

6. Former NIH legislative aide Marc Smolonsky.

7. Former NIH legislative aide Marc Smolonsky.

8. Former NIH legislative aide Marc Smolonsky.

9. Former NIH legislative aide Marc Smolonsky.

10. Former NIH legislative aide Marc Smolonsky.

11. Former NIH legislative aide Marc Smolonsky.

12. Elias Zerhouni, "A Statement from the NIH Director, Elias A. Zerhouni, MD, regarding the 'National Institutes of Health Reform Act of 2006,'" NIH, December 10, 2006, https://www.nih.gov/about-nih/who-we-are/nih-director/statements/statement-nih-director-elias-zerhouni-md-regarding-national-institutes-health-reform-act-2006.

13. Zerhouni, "The NIH Reform Act of 2006."

14. Zerhouni, "The NIH Reform Act of 2006."

15. Zerhouni, "The NIH Reform Act of 2006."

16. Zerhouni, "The NIH Reform Act of 2006."

17. Zerhouni, "The NIH Reform Act of 2006."

18. Jeremy Berg, notes to the author, July 22, 2024.

19. Jeremy Berg, notes to the author, July 22, 2024.

20. "NIH Director Announces Enhancements to Peer Review," news releases, NIH, June 6, 2008, https://www.nih.gov/news-events/news-releases/nih-director-announces-enhancements-peer-review.

21. "NIH Director Announces Enhancements to Peer Review."

22. Megan Scudellari, "How iPS Cells Changed the World," *Nature* 534 (2016): 310–12, https://doi.org/10.1038/534310a; "Shinya Yamanaka," Nobel

Prize in Physiology or Medicine 2012, accessed September 9, 2023, https://www.nobelprize.org/prizes/medicine/2012/yamanaka/facts.

23. "Shinya Yamanaka," Nobel Prize in Physiology or Medicine 2012, accessed September 9, 2023, https://www.nobelprize.org/prizes/medicine/2012/yamanaka/facts.

24. Martin Fackler, "Risk Taking Is in His Genes," *New York Times*, December 11, 2007, https://www.nytimes.com/2007/12/11/science/11prof.html.

25. Natalie Lamont, e-mail to the author, October 23, 2024.

26. "NIH Director Nomination," C-Span, April 30, 2002, https://www.c-span.org/video/?169822-1/nih-director-nomination.

27. Lisa Stein, "NIH Chief Calls for More Stem Cell Research," *Scientific American*, March 20, 2007, https://www.scientificamerican.com/article/nih-chief-calls-for-more.

28. Stein, "NIH Chief Calls for More Stem Cell Research."

29. "Advancing Stem Cell Research in Ethical, Responsible Ways," White House Archives of President George W. Bush, accessed October 31, 2024, https://georgewbush-whitehouse.archives.gov/infocus/bushrecord/factsheets/stemcells.html.

30. "Advancing Stem Cell Research in Ethical, Responsible Ways."

31. "Advancing Stem Cell Research in Ethical, Responsible Ways."

32. Dr. Howard Markel, "How the Discovery of HIV Led to a Transatlantic Research War," *PBS NewsHour*, PBS, March 24, 2020, https://www.pbs.org/newshour/health/how-the-discovery-of-hiv-led-to-a-transatlantic-research-war.

33. Markel, "How the Discovery of HIV Led to a Transatlantic Research War."

34. Randi Hutter Epstein, "Luc Montagnier, Nobel-Winning Co-Discoverer of H.I.V., Dies at 89," *New York Times*, February 10, 2022, https://www.nytimes.com/2022/02/10/science/luc-montagnier-dead.html; Markel, "How the Discovery of HIV Led to a Transatlantic Research War."

35. Edwin Chen, "U.S. Admits French Role in HIV Test Kit: Health: Officials Say That the Virus Used by Scientists Came from France. Royalties Will Be More Evenly Split under a New Agreement," *Los Angeles Times*, July 12, 1994, https://www.latimes.com/archives/la-xpm-1994-07-12-mn-14822-story.html.

36. Chen, "U.S. Admits French Role in HIV Test Kit."

37. Chen, "U.S. Admits French Role in HIV Test Kit."

38. Chen, "U.S. Admits French Role in HIV Test Kit."

39. Martin Enserink, "Will French Science Swallow Zerhouni's Strong Medicine?," *Science* 322, no. 5906 (2008): 1312, https://doi.org/10.1126/science.322.5906.1312.

40. Enserink, "Will French Science Swallow Zerhouni's Strong Medicine?"

41. "Elias A. Zerhouni, MD," The NIH Almanac, NIH, last reviewed on October 22, 2015, https://www.nih.gov/about-nih/what-we-do/nih-almanac/elias-zerhouni-md.

Chapter 21. Legion of Honour, the Gates Foundation, and Becoming a Presidential Envoy

1. "Elias Zerhouni, MD, Joins Foundation—Bill & Melinda Gates Foundation," Bill & Melinda Gates Foundation, accessed August 25, 2023, https://www.gatesfoundation.org/ideas/media-center/press-releases/2009/02/elias-zerhouni-md-joins-foundation-as-a-senior-fellow.

2. "About Grand Challenges Initiatives," Grand Challenges, accessed August 17, 2023, https://www.grandchallenges.org/about.

3. "The President's Speech in Cairo: A New Beginning," The White House of President Barack Obama, accessed August 25, 2023, https://obamawhitehouse.archives.gov/issues/foreign-policy/presidents-speech-cairo-a-new-beginning.

4. "Remarks by the President at Cairo University, 6-04-09," Office of the Press Secretary, The White House of President Barack Obama, June 4, 2009, https://obamawhitehouse.archives.gov/the-press-office/remarks-president-cairo-university-6-04-09.

5. Harold Varmus, e-mail to the author, July 27, 2024.

6. Elias Zerhouni, "Episode 16: Elias Zerhouni, MD, FACR," interviewed by Geoff Rubin, Taking the Lead, Radiology Leadership Institute, December 19, 2019, transcript, https://www.acr.org/-/media/ACR/Files/RLI/Podcasts/Ep-16-Zerhouni_TranscriptFinal.pdf.

7. "Three New Science Envoys Announced," The White House of President Barack Obama, September 17, 2010, https://obamawhitehouse.archives.gov/blog/2010/09/17/three-new-science-envoys-announced.

8. Elias Zerhouni, "Space for the Cures: Science Launches a New Journal Dedicated to Translational Research in Biomedicine," *Science Translational Medicine* 1, no. 1 (2009): 1, https://doi.org/10.1126/scitranslmed.3000341.

9. Zerhouni, "Space for the Cures."
10. Zerhouni, "Space for the Cures."
11. Zerhouni, "Space for the Cures."
12. Zerhouni, "Space for the Cures."
13. Zerhouni, "Space for the Cures."
14. *Science Translational Medicine, Science*, accessed August 25, 2023, https://www.science.org/content/page/stm-information-authors.
15. Zerhouni, "Space for the Cures."
16. Jim Greenwood, e-mail to the author, July 21, 2024.

Chapter 22. Sanofi

1. Reuters Staff, "Factbox: Key Facts about Sanofi and Genzyme," Reuters, February 16, 2011, https://www.reuters.com/article/us-sanofi-genzyme-facts-idUSTRE71F1K320110216.

2. Ransdell Pierson, "Genzyme Discards Drugs due to One-Time Problems," Reuters, August 11, 2010, https://www.reuters.com/article/us-genzyme-idUK TRE67A20Q20100811.

3. Matthew Herper, "Pharma's Missing Link," Forbes, June 6, 2012, https:// www.forbes.com/forbes/2012/0625/strategies-elias-zerhouni-sanofi-pharma -missing-link.html.

4. Richard K. Harrison and Laura J. Vitez, "Strategic Trends in Big Pharma Dealmaking," Biopharma Dealmakers, Nature, June 9, 2017, https://www.nature .com/articles/d43747-020-00317-8.

5. Herper, "Pharma's Missing Link."

6. "Sanofi and Warp Drive Bio to Collaborate on the Development of Novel Oncology Therapies and Antibiotics Based on Proprietary Platforms," Business Wire, January 11, 2016, https://www.businesswire.com/news/home/201601100 05026/en/Sanofi-Warp-Drive-Bio-Collaborate-Development-Oncology.

7. Herper, "Pharma's Missing Link."

8. Herper, "Pharma's Missing Link."

9. Herper, "Pharma's Missing Link."

10. Herper, "Pharma's Missing Link."

11. "Sanofi and MyoKardia Announce Groundbreaking Collaboration to Develop Targeted Therapies for Patients with Genetic Heart Disease," Sanofi, September 17, 2014, https://www.news.sanofi.us/2014-09-17-Sanofi-and-Myo Kardia-Announce-Groundbreaking-Collaboration-to-Develop-Targeted-Thera pies-for-Patients-with-Genetic-Heart-Disease.

12. "Sanofi and MyoKardia Announce Groundbreaking Collaboration to De-velop Targeted Therapies for Patients with Genetic Heart Disease."

13. "Bristol Myers Squibb to Acquire MyoKardia for $13.1 Billion in Cash," Bristol-Myers Squibb, October 5, 2020, https://news.bms.com/news/de tails/2020/Bristol-Myers-Squibb-to-Acquire-MyoKardia-for-13.1-Billion-in -Cash/default.aspx.

14. Noëlle Mennella, "Sanofi to Cut 207 R&D Jobs in Latest French Re-shuffle," Reuters, July 2, 2013, https://www.reuters.com/article/us-sanofi-rd -idUKBRE9610WC20130702.

15. "Elias Zerhouni, President of Sanofi R&D, Wins 'Executive of the Year' at Annual Scrip Awards," press release, Sanofi, November 30, 2017, https://www .sanofi.com/assets/dotcom/pressreleases/2017/2017-11-30-06-55-03-1211688 -en.pdf.

16. "Elias Zerhouni, President of Sanofi R&D, Wins 'Executive of the Year' at Annual Scrip Awards."

17. "Elias Zerhouni, President of Sanofi R&D, Wins 'Executive of the Year' at Annual Scrip Awards."

Chapter 23. Unretirement and ModeX

1. Lasker Foundation, accessed August 27, 2023, https://laskerfoundation.org/about-us/mission.

2. Lasker Foundation.

3. John Hardy and Dennis J. Selkoe, "The Amyloid Hypothesis of Alzheimer's Disease: Progress and Problems on the Road to Therapeutics," *Science* 297, no. 5580 (2002): 353–56, https://doi.org/10.1126/science.1072994.

4. "Dementia Experts Meet in Lausanne to Discuss Alzheimer's Diagnosis," Alzheimer Europe, November 13, 2019, https://www.alzheimer-europe.org/news/dementia-experts-meet-lausanne-discuss-alzheimers-diagnosis.

5. "Our Beginning," Davos Alzheimer's Collaborative, accessed August 27, 2023, https://www.davosalzheimerscollaborative.org.

6. Elias Zerhouni, "Former NIH Director Dr. Elias Zerhouni | Breaking New Ground: Innovations in Alzheimer's Research," interviewed by Steve Clemons, The Hill Events, The Hill, March 2, 2022, video, https://www.youtube.com/watch?v=JUdsK4Bt3f8.

7. "About Us," Davos Alzheimer's Collaborative, accessed August 27, 2023, https://www.davosalzheimerscollaborative.org.

8. "About Us."

9. "The Challenge," Leading an Unprecedented Global Response to Alzheimer's, Davos Alzheimer's Collaborative, accessed August 27, 2023, https://www.davosalzheimerscollaborative.org.

10. "The Challenge."

11. "The Challenge."

12. "Waypoint Capital Appoints Elias Zerhouni to Board of Directors," Business Wire, August 27, 2023, https://www.businesswire.com/news/home/20200108005148/en/Waypoint-Capital-Appoints-Elias-Zerhouni-Board-Directors.

13. Dan Diamond and Adam Cancryn, "Former NIH Chief Favored as Trump's 'Therapeutics Czar,'" *Politico*, May 8, 2020, https://www.politico.com/news/2020/05/08/former-nih-chief-zerhouni-favored-as-trumps-therapeutics-czar-245631.

14. Joe Palca, "Former NIH Director Calls Trump Administration's Pandemic Response 'Amateur Hour,'" NPR, June 29, 2020, https://www.npr.org/sections/health-shots/2020/06/29/884435625/former-nih-director-calls-trump-administrations-pandemic-response-amateur-hour.

15. Palca, "Former NIH Director Calls Trump Administration's Pandemic Response 'Amateur Hour.'"

16. Palca, "Former NIH Director Calls Trump Administration's Pandemic Response 'Amateur Hour.'"

17. Palca, "Former NIH Director Calls Trump Administration's Pandemic Response 'Amateur Hour.'"

18. Palca, "Former NIH Director Calls Trump Administration's Pandemic Response 'Amateur Hour.'"

19. "OPKO Health Acquires ModeX Therapeutics, Gains Proprietary Immunotherapy Technology with a Focus on Oncology and Infectious Diseases," press releases, OPKO, May 9, 2022, https://www.opko.com/news-media/press-releases/detail/467/opko-health-acquires-modex-therapeutics-gains-proprietary.

20. "OPKO Health Acquires ModeX Therapeutics, Gains Proprietary Immunotherapy Technology with a Focus on Oncology and Infectious Diseases"; "NIH Launches Clinical Trial of Epstein-Barr Virus Vaccine," news releases, NIH, May 6, 2022, https://www.nih.gov/news-events/news-releases/nih-launches-clinical-trial-epstein-barr-virus-vaccine.

21. "OPKO Health's ModeX Therapeutics Enters into Exclusive Worldwide License and Collaboration Agreement with Merck to Develop Epstein-Barr Virus Vaccine Candidate," press releases, OPKO, March 8, 2023, https://www.opko.com/investors/news-events/press-releases/detail/478/opko-healths-modex-therapeutics-enters-into-exclusive.

Chapter 24. Lessons, Science, Immigration, and America

1. A Manichean is, quite literally, "a believer in a syncretistic religious dualism originating in Persia in the third century AD and teaching the release of the spirit from matter through asceticism" (https://www.merriam-webster.com/dictionary/Manichaean). In this case, I'm using the term in a colloquial sense as an adjective to describe a black-and-white way of thinking.

Bibliography

Abell Foundation. "Our Commitment." Accessed August 5, 2024. https://abell
.org.

"About Grand Challenges Initiatives." Grand Challenges. Accessed August 17,
2023. https://www.grandchallenges.org/about.

"About Us." Davos Alzheimer's Collaborative. Accessed August 27, 2023.
https://www.davosalzheimerscollaborative.org.

"Advancing Stem Cell Research in Ethical, Responsible Ways." White House
Archives of President George W. Bush. Accessed October 31, 2024. https://
georgewbush-whitehouse.archives.gov/infocus/bushrecord/factsheets/stem
cells.html.

"Algerian War: Macron in Rare Torture Admission." BBC. September 13, 2018.
https://www.bbc.com/news/world-europe-45513842.

"Amerithrax or Anthrax Investigation." History, FBI. Accessed August 17, 2023.
www.fbi.gov/history/famous-cases/amerithrax-or-anthrax-investigation.

Baer, Susan. "NIH Chief Balancing Politics and Science." *Baltimore Sun.* May
2, 2005. https://www.baltimoresun.com/news/bs-xpm-2005-05-02-0505020
010-story.html.

Beck, Andrew H. "The Flexner Report and the Standardization of American
Medical Education." *Journal of the American Medical Association* 291, no. 17
(2004): 2139–40. https://doi.org/10.1001/jama.291.17.2139.

Bradley, Ryan. "This Is Your Brain on . . . Surgical Sound Waves." *Fortune.* June
12, 2014. https://fortune.com/2014/06/12/focused-ultrasound-surgery.

"Bristol Myers Squibb to Acquire MyoKardia for $13.1 Billion in Cash." Bristol-
Myers Squibb. October 5, 2020. https://news.bms.com/news/details/2020
/Bristol-Myers-Squibb-to-Acquire-MyoKardia-for-13.1-Billion-in-Cash/de
fault.aspx.

Cazier, Crystal, and Andrew Kaufmann. "An Oral History of PEPFAR: How
a 'Dream Big' Partnership Is Saving the Lives of Millions." George W. Bush

Presidential Center. February 24, 2023. https://www.bushcenter.org/publi
cations/an-oral-history-of-pepfar-how-a-dream-big-partnership-is-saving-the
-lives-of-millions.

Check, Erika. "Ethics Accusations Spark Rapid Reaction from NIH Chief." *Nature* 427, no. 187 (2004). https://doi.org/10.1038/427187b.

Chen, Edwin. "U.S. Admits French Role in HIV Test Kit: Health: Officials Say
That the Virus Used by Scientists Came from France. Royalties Will Be More
Evenly Split under a New Agreement." *Los Angeles Times.* July 12, 1994. https://
www.latimes.com/archives/la-xpm-1994-07-12-mn-14822-story.html.

"Dementia Experts Meet in Lausanne to Discuss Alzheimer's Diagnosis." Alzheimer Europe. November 13, 2019. https://www.alzheimer-europe.org/news
/dementia-experts-meet-lausanne-discuss-alzheimers-diagnosis.

Diamond, Dan, and Adam Cancryn. "Former NIH Chief Favored as Trump's
'Therapeutics Czar.'" *Politico.* May 8, 2020. https://www.politico.com/news
/2020/05/08/former-nih-chief-zerhouni-favored-as-trumps-therapeutics
-czar-245631.

Duffy, Thomas P. "The Flexner Report—100 Years Later." *Yale Journal of Biology
and Medicine* 84, no. 3 (2011): 269–76. https://www.ncbi.nlm.nih.gov/pmc
/articles/PMC3178858.

Dunn, Kyla. "The Politics of Stem Cells." PBS. April 1, 2005. https://www.pbs
.org/wgbh/nova/article/stem-cells-politics.

"E. Robert Heitzman, MD, Former RSNA President, Dies at 93." RSNA News.
Radiological Society of North America. November 12, 2020. https://www
.rsna.org/news/2020/october/in-memoriam-robert-heitzman#.

Editorial. "Rethinking Grant Review." *Nature Neuroscience* 11, no. 2 (2008): 119.
https://www.nature.com/articles/nn0208-119.pdf.

Educational Commission for Foreign Medical Graduates. "History." Last updated
February 10, 2023. https://www.ecfmg.org/about/history.html.

"Elias A. Zerhouni, MD." The NIH Almanac, NIH. Last reviewed October
22, 2015. https://www.nih.gov/about-nih/what-we-do/nih-almanac/elias
-zerhouni-md.

"Elias Zerhouni, MD, Joins Foundation—Bill & Melinda Gates Foundation." Bill & Melinda Gates Foundation. Accessed August 25, 2023. https://
www.gatesfoundation.org/ideas/media-center/press-releases/2009/02/elias
-zerhouni-md-joins-foundation-as-a-senior-fellow.

"Elias A. Zerhouni, MD, Radiologist: New Director of the National Institutes
of Health." *Radiology* 224, no. 2 (2002): 309. https://doi.org/10.1148/radiol
.2242020547.

"Elias Zerhouni, President of Sanofi R&D, Wins 'Executive of the Year' at
Annual Scrip Awards." Press release. Sanofi. November 30, 2017. https://
www.sanofi.com/assets/dotcom/pressreleases/2017/2017-11-30-06-55-03
-1211688-en.pdf.

Enserink, Martin. "Will French Science Swallow Zerhouni's Strong Medicine?" *Science* 322, no. 5906 (2008): 1312. https://doi.org/10.1126/science.322.5906.1312.

Epstein, Randi Hutter. "Luc Montagnier, Nobel-Winning Co-Discoverer of H.I.V., Dies at 89." *New York Times*. February 10, 2022. https://www.nytimes.com/2022/02/10/science/luc-montagnier-dead.html.

Fackler, Martin. "Risk Taking Is in His Genes." *New York Times*. December 11, 2007. https://www.nytimes.com/2007/12/11/science/11prof.html.

"'Father of Modern Medicine': The Johns Hopkins School of Medicine, 1889–1905." National Library of Medicine Profiles in Science. NIH. Accessed August 28, 2023. https://profiles.nlm.nih.gov/spotlight/gf/feature/father-of-modern-medicine-the-johns-hopkins-school-of-medicine-1889-1905.

Fauci, Anthony S., and Robert W. Eisinger. "PEPFAR—15 Years and Counting the Lives Saved." *New England Journal of Medicine* 378 (2018): 314–16. https://doi.org/10.1056/NEJMp1714773.

"Fourteen Grand Challenges in Global Health Announced in $200 Million Initiative." Bill & Melinda Gates Foundation. Accessed August 17, 2023. https://www.gatesfoundation.org/Ideas/Media-Center/Press-Releases/2003/10/14-Grand-Challenges-in-Global-Health.

Good, I. J. *The Scientist Speculates*. New York: Basic Books, 1962.

Grady, Denise. "A Conversation with: Elias Zerhouni; Learning the Science of Leading." *New York Times*. July 15, 2003. https://www.nytimes.com/2003/07/15/science/a-conversation-with-elias-zerhouni-learning-the-science-of-leading.html.

Hardy, John, and Dennis J. Selkoe. "The Amyloid Hypothesis of Alzheimer's Disease: Progress and Problems on the Road to Therapeutics." *Science* 297, no. 5580 (2002): 353–56. https://doi.org/10.1126/science.1072994.

Harrison, Richard K., and Laura J. Vitez. "Strategic Trends in Big Pharma Dealmaking." Biopharma Dealmakers. *Nature*. June 9, 2017. https://www.nature.com/articles/d43747-020-00317-8.

Häusser, Michael. "Optogenetics—The Might of Light." *New England Journal of Medicine* 385 (2021): 1623–26. https://doi.org/10.1056/NEJMcibr2111915.

Herper, Matthew. "Pharma's Missing Link." *Forbes*. June 6, 2012. https://www.forbes.com/forbes/2012/0625/strategies-elias-zerhouni-sanofi-pharma-missing-link.html.

Higgins, Edmund S. "Fifty Years Ago, the First CT Scan Let Doctors See inside a Living Skull." *Smithsonian Magazine*. October 1, 2021. https://www.smithsonianmag.com/innovation/fifty-years-ago-the-first-ct-scan-let-doctors-see-inside-a-living-skull-180978792.

Hitchens, Christopher. "A Chronology of the Algerian War of Independence." *The Atlantic*. November 2006. https://www.theatlantic.com/magazine/archive/2006/11/a-chronology-of-the-algerian-war-of-independence/305277.

Horne, Alistair. *A Savage War of Peace: Algeria 1954–1962*. New York: New York Review Books, 2011. Kindle.

Kaiser, Jocelyn. "NIH Roiled by Inquiries over Grants Hit List." *Science* 302, no. 5646 (2003): 758. https://doi.org/10.1126/science.302.5646.758.

———. "NIH Urged to Focus on New Ideas, New Applicants." *Science* 319, no. 5867 (2008): 1169. https://doi.org/10.1126/science.319.5867.1169.

———. "Sex Studies 'Properly' Approved." *Science* 303, no. 5659 (2004): 741. https://doi.org/10.1126/science.303.5659.741a.

———. "Zerhouni Confirmed as NIH Director." *Science* 296, no. 5570 (2002): 997–99. https://doi.org/10.1126/science.296.5570.997b.

"Key Moments in the Stem-Cell Debate." NPR. November 20, 2007. https://www.npr.org/templates/story/story.php?storyId=5252449.

Kimmelman, Michael. "Footprints of Pieds-Noirs Reach Deep into France." *New York Times*. March 5, 2009. https://www.nytimes.com/2009/03/05/world/europe/05iht-kimmel.4.20622745.html.

Knight, Jonathan. "Accusations of Bias Prompt NIH Review of Ethical Guidelines." *Nature* 426, no. 741 (2003). https://doi.org/10.1038/426741a.

Koenig, Sarah, and David Nitkin. "Howard 'Pete' Rawlings Dies at 66." *Baltimore Sun*. November 14, 2003. https://msa.maryland.gov/megafile/msa/speccol/sc3500/sc3520/012200/012298/html/sun14nov2003.html.

Kozel, Peter. "NIH's Roadmap to the Future." *Science*. Published January 9, 2004. https://doi.org/10.1126/article.65945.

Lang, Les. "NIH Weighs Peer Review Changes." *Gastroenterology* 134, no. 2 (2008): 380. https://doi.org/10.1053/j.gastro.2007.12.040.

Lasker Foundation. Accessed August 27, 2023. https://laskerfoundation.org/about-us/mission.

Markel, Howard. "How the Discovery of HIV Led to a Transatlantic Research War." PBS NewsHour. PBS. March 24, 2020. https://www.pbs.org/newshour/health/how-the-discovery-of-hiv-led-to-a-transatlantic-research-war.

McAuley, James. "France's Macron Admits to Military's Systematic Use of Torture in Algeria War." *Washington Post*. September 13, 2018. https://www.washingtonpost.com/world/europe/frances-macron-admits-to-militarys-systematic-use-of-torture-in-algeria-war/2018/09/13/6b0e85cc-b729-11e8-94eb-3bd52dfe917b_story.html.

———. "In France, a 1961 Massacre Looms Large behind a Controversial New Law." *Washington Post*. October 20, 2017. https://www.washingtonpost.com/world/europe/in-france-a-1961-massacre-looms-large-behind-a-controversial-new-law/2017/10/20/82a95e7c-b334-11e7-9b93-b97043e57a22_story.html.

McDougall, James. *A History of Algeria*. Cambridge: Cambridge University Press, 2017. Kindle.

Mennella, Noëlle. "Sanofi to Cut 207 R&D Jobs in Latest French Reshuffle." Reuters. July 2, 2013. https://www.reuters.com/article/us-sanofi-rd-idUKBRE9610WC20130702.

"NIH Director Announces Enhancements to Peer Review." News releases. NIH. June 6, 2008. https://www.nih.gov/news-events/news-releases/nih-director-an nounces-enhancements-peer-review.

"NIH Director Nomination." C-Span. Filmed April 30, 2002. https://www .c-span.org/video/?169822-1/nih-director-nomination.

"NIH Director's Pioneer Award Recipients, 2005 Awardees." NIH Director's Pioneer Award. NIH. Last reviewed July 23, 2021. https://commonfund.nih .gov/pioneer/AwardRecipients05.

NIH Ethics Concerns: Consulting Arrangements and Outside Awards; Hearings before the Subcommittee on Oversight and Investigations of the Committee on Energy and Commerce House of Representatives; One Hundred Eighth Congress, Second Session, May 12, May 18, and June 22, 2004. Washington, DC: U.S. Government Printing Office. 2004.

"NIH Launches Clinical Trial of Epstein-Barr Virus Vaccine." News releases. NIH. May 6, 2022. https://www.nih.gov/news-events/news-releases/nih -launches-clinical-trial-epstein-barr-virus-vaccine.

"NIH Working Group on Women in Biomedical Careers." NIH. Accessed August 25, 2023. https://orwh.od.nih.gov/career-development-education/nih-working -group-on-women-in-biomedical-careers.

Office of NIH History, Office of Communications and Public Liaison, and Office of the Director. *NIH Events 2003–2004, Elias A. Zerhouni, MD, Director* (2003–2004).

———. *NIH Events 2004–2005, Elias A. Zerhouni, MD, Director* (2004–2005).

———. *NIH Events 2005–2006, Elias A. Zerhouni, MD, Director* (2005–2006).

O'Grady, Siobhan. "As Algeria's Revolutionaries Fade Away, the Iconic Milk Bar Bomber Looks Back without Regret." *Washington Post.* July 9, 2021. https:// www.washingtonpost.com/world/middle_east/algeria-france--zohra-drif -milk-bar/2021/07/08/7f788f6c-d5c6-11eb-b39f-05a2d776b1f4_story.html.

"OPKO Health Acquires ModeX Therapeutics, Gains Proprietary Immunotherapy Technology with a Focus on Oncology and Infectious Diseases." Press releases. OPKO. May 9, 2022. https://www.opko.com/news-media/press-re leases/detail/467/opko-health-acquires-modex-therapeutics-gains-proprietary.

"OPKO Health's ModeX Therapeutics Enters into Exclusive Worldwide License and Collaboration Agreement with Merck to Develop Epstein-Barr Virus Vaccine Candidate." Press releases. OPKO. March 8, 2023. https://www.opko .com/investors/news-events/press-releases/detail/478/opko-healths-modex -therapeutics-enters-into-exclusive.

Ortiz, Fiona, and Justin Madden. "Ex-House Speaker Hastert Gets 15 Months, Admits Sex Abuse." Reuters. April 27, 2016. https://www.reuters.com/ar ticle/us-crime-hastert-idUSKCN0XO178.

"Our Beginning." Davos Alzheimer's Collaborative. Accessed August 27, 2023. https://www.davosalzheimerscollaborative.org.

Palca, Joe. "Former NIH Director Calls Trump Administration's Pandemic Response 'Amateur Hour.'" NPR. June 29, 2020. https://www.npr.org/sections/health-shots/2020/06/29/884435625/former-nih-director-calls-trump-administrations-pandemic-response-amateur hour.

"Pandemic and All Hazards Preparedness Act (PAHPA)." Administration for Strategic Preparedness and Response. HHS.gov. Accessed August 17, 2023. https://www.phe.gov/preparedness/legal/pahpa/pages/default.aspx.

Pierson, Ransdell. "Genzyme Discards Drugs due to One-Time Problems." Reuters. August 11, 2010. https://www.reuters.com/article/us-genzyme-idUKTRE67A20Q20100811.

Pinholster, Ginger. "Bruce Alberts, Elias Zerhouni and Ahmed Zewail Named First U.S. Science Envoys." American Association for the Advancement of Science. November 5, 2009. https://www.aaas.org/news/bruce-alberts-elias-zerhouni-and-ahmed-zewail-named-first-us-science-envoys.

"President Nominates NIH Director and Surgeon General." Office of the Press Secretary. White House Archives of President George W. Bush. March 26, 2002. https://georgewbush-whitehouse.archives.gov/news/releases/2002/03/20020326-3.html.

"Remarks by the President at Cairo University, 6-04-09." Office of the Press Secretary. White House of President Barack Obama. June 4, 2009. https://obamawhitehouse.archives.gov/the-press-office/remarks-president-cairo-university-6-04-09.

Research!America. Accessed August 27, 2023. https://www.researchamerica.org/who-we-are.

Reuters Staff. "Factbox: Key Facts about Sanofi and Genzyme." Reuters. February 16, 2011. https://www.reuters.com/article/us-sanofi-genzyme-facts-idUSTRE71F1K320110216.

Rienzi, Greg. "Biotech Park to Rise in East Baltimore." *The Gazette*. April 22, 2002. https://pages.jh.edu/gazette/2002/22apr02/22biotec.html.

"S.3678—Pandemic and All-Hazards Preparedness Act." 109th Congress (2005–2006). Congress.gov. Accessed August 17, 2023. https://www.congress.gov/bill/109th-congress/senate-bill/3678.

Salganik, M. William. "JH Medical Selects Chief Financial Officer Grossi Is Promoted by Entity Now Overseeing Med School, Health System." *Baltimore Sun*. August 31, 2023. https://www.baltimoresun.com/news/bs-xpm-1996-09-21-1996265088-story.html.

"Sanofi and MyoKardia Announce Groundbreaking Collaboration to Develop Targeted Therapies for Patients with Genetic Heart Disease." Sanofi. September 17, 2014. https://www.news.sanofi.us/2014-09-17-Sanofi-and-MyoKardia-Announce-Groundbreaking-Collaboration-to-Develop-Targeted-Therapies-for-Patients-with-Genetic-Heart-Disease.

"Sanofi and Warp Drive Bio to Collaborate on the Development of Novel Oncology Therapies and Antibiotics Based on Proprietary Platforms." Business Wire. Jan-

uary 11, 2016. https://www.businesswire.com/news/home/20160110005026
/en/Sanofi-Warp-Drive-Bio-Collaborate-Development-Oncology.

Schudel, Matt. "Louis P. Sheldon, Inflammatory Anti-Gay Crusader of 'Traditional Values,' Dies at 85." *Washington Post*. June 6, 2020. https://www
.washingtonpost.com/local/obituaries/louis-p-sheldon-inflammatory-anti-gay
-crusader-of-traditional-values-dies-at-85/2020/06/06/20fcb81a-a80d-11ea
-bb20-ebf0921f3bbd_story.html.

Science Translational Medicine. Science. Accessed August 25, 2023. https://www.sci
ence.org/content/page/stm-information-authors.

Scudellari, Megan. "How iPS Cells Changed the World." *Nature* 534 (2016):
310–12. https://doi.org/10.1038/534310a.

Sekar, Kavya. "National Institutes of Health (NIH) Funding: FY1996-FY2024."
Congressional Research Service. Updated May 17, 2023. https://sgp.fas.org
/crs/misc/R43341.pdf.

"Shake-Up at Johns Hopkins Dr. Block's Departure: Medical School, Hospital under New Leaders and New Structure." *Baltimore Sun*. August 11, 1996. https://
www.baltimoresun.com/news/bs-xpm-1996-08-11-1996224012-story.html.

"Shinya Yamanaka." Nobel Prize in Physiology or Medicine 2012. Accessed
September 9, 2023. https://www.nobelprize.org/prizes/medicine/2012/ya-
manaka/facts.

Stein, Lisa. "Bush Vetoes Stem Cell Bill; Lawmakers Offer New One." *Scientific
American*. June 22, 2007. https://www.scientificamerican.com/article/bush-ve
toes-stem-cell-bill.

———. "NIH Chief Calls for More Stem Cell Research." *Scientific American*.
March 20, 2007. https://www.scientificamerican.com/article/nih-chief-calls
-for-more.

Steinbrook, Robert. "Financial Conflicts of Interest and the NIH." *New England Journal of Medicine* 350 (2004): 327–30. https://doi.org/10.1056/NEJMp
038247.

"Sunshine Act." Johns Hopkins University & Medicine. Last updated November
2022. https://industryinteraction.jhu.edu/sunshine-act.

"Surgeon General Nomination." C-Span. Filmed March 26, 2002. https://
www.c-span.org/video/?169340-1/surgeon-general-nomination.

"The President's Speech in Cairo: A New Beginning." The White House of
President Barack Obama. Accessed August 25, 2023. https://obamawhitehouse
.archives.gov/issues/foreign-policy/presidents-speech-cairo-a-new-beginning.

"Three New Science Envoys Announced." The White House of President
Barack Obama. September 17, 2010. https://obamawhitehouse.archives.gov
/blog/2010/09/17/three-new-science-envoys-announced.

"Timeline: How the Anthrax Terror Unfolded." *The Anthrax Investigation*. NPR.
February 15, 2011. https://www.npr.org/2011/02/15/93170200/timeline-how
-the-anthrax-terror-unfolded.

UPI. "Andres Gruentzig Dies in Air Crash." *New York Times*. October 29, 1985. https://www.nytimes.com/1985/10/29/us/andres-gruentzig-dies-in-air-crash.html.

Varmus, H., R. Klausner, E. Zerhouni, T. Acharya, A. S. Daar, and P. A. Singer. "Grand Challenges in Global Health." *Science* 302, no. 5644 (2003): 398–99. https://doi.org/10.1126/science.1091769.

Wadman, Meredith. "Early Success Claimed for Zerhouni's NIH Roadmap." *Nature* 431, no. 886 (2004). https://doi.org/10.1038/431886b.

"Waypoint Capital Appoints Elias Zerhouni to Board of Directors." Business Wire. August 27, 2023. https://www.businesswire.com/news/home/20200108005148/en/Waypoint-Capital-Appoints-Elias-Zerhouni-Board-Directors.

Wehner, Peter. "My Friend, Mike Gerson." *The Atlantic*. November 18, 2022. https://www.theatlantic.com/ideas/archive/2022/11/michael-gerson-speech writer-george-bush-dies-cancer/672172.

Weiss, Rick. "NIH to Fund Controversial Research." *Washington Post*. January 20, 1999. https://www.washingtonpost.com/wp-srv/national/daily/jan99/stemcells20.htm.

"Who We Are." NIH. Accessed August 1, 2024. https://www.nih.gov/about-nih/who-we-are.

Willman, David. "Stealth Merger: Drug Companies and Government Medical Research." *Los Angeles Times*. December 7, 2003. https://www.latimes.com/archives/la-xpm-2003-dec-07-na-nih7-story.html.

Willman, David, and Jon Marino. "NIH Directors No Longer Drug Firm Consultants." *Los Angeles Times*. January 23, 2004. https://www.latimes.com/archives/la-xpm-2004-jan-23-na-nih23-story.html.

Zerhouni, Elias. "Episode 16: Elias Zerhouni, MD, FACR." Interviewed by Geoff Rubin. Taking the Lead, Radiology Leadership Institute. December 19, 2019. Transcript. https://www.acr.org/-/media/ACR/Files/RLI/Podcasts/Ep-16-Zerhouni_TranscriptFinal.pdf.

———. "Former NIH Director Dr. Elias Zerhouni | Breaking New Ground: Innovations in Alzheimer's Research." Interviewed by Steve Clemons. The Hill Events. The Hill. March 2, 2022. Video. https://www.youtube.com/watch?v=JUdsK4Bt3f8.

———. "The NIH Reform Act of 2006: Progress, Challenges, and Next Steps." News releases. NIH. Published September 9, 2008. https://www.nih.gov/news-events/news-releases/nih-reform-act-2006-progress-challenges-next-steps.

———. "The NIH Roadmap." *Science* 302, no. 5642 (2003): 63–72. https://doi.org/10.1126/science.1091867.

———. "Opening Statement Senate Hearings Elias A. Zerhouni, MD, Director-Nominee- NIH." HELP Committee, U.S. Senate. Accessed August 8, 2023. https://www.help.senate.gov/imo/media/doc/Zerhouni2.pdf.

———. "Space for the Cures: Science Launches a New Journal Dedicated to Translational Research in Biomedicine." *Science Translational Medicine* 1, no. 1 (2009): 1. https://doi.org/10.1126/scitranslmed.3000341.

———. "A Statement from the NIH Director, Elias A. Zerhouni, MD, regarding the 'National Institutes of Health Reform Act of 2006.'" NIH. December 10, 2006. https://www.nih.gov/about-nih/who-we-are/nih-director/statements/statement-nih-director-elias-zerhouni-md-regarding-national-institutes-health-reform-act-2006.

Zerhouni, E. A., F. P. Stitik, S. S. Siegelman, D. P. Naidich, S. S. Sagel, A. V. Proto, J. R. Muhm, J. W. Walsh, C. R. Martinez, R. T. Heelan, et al. "CT of the Pulmonary Nodule: A Cooperative Study." *Radiology* 160 (1986): 319–27. https://doi.org/10.1148/radiology.160.2.3726107.

Acknowledgments

I'd like to acknowledge all those who helped with the memoir's creation. First and foremost, I thank my wife, Nadia, for supporting me in this project and spending many hours reviewing text and pictures and aiding my recollection of our shared past. Meanwhile, my longtime friend Bruce Holbrook tirelessly dedicated himself to this project, advising me as I brought my life story to the page. Bruce first suggested the idea of the memoir back in the early 2010s. From that moment on, he kept pushing me to write this book. Eventually, I acquiesced and enlisted the services of Edward Kriz to assist me as I crafted the manuscript.

I'd like to thank Jonathan Kurtz, executive editor of Prometheus Books, for taking on this project. It speaks volumes about his upstanding values and boldness; his publishing company, Prometheus Books; and their owner, Globe Pequot. Jonathan and his supporting staff, including Brianna Soubannarath, Chloe Hummel, Nicole Myers, Bruce Owens, and Annette Van Deusen, are exceptional, and they provided invaluable support throughout. I am honored to have *Disease Knows No Politics* be a part of Prometheus Books' impactful, transformative catalog.

In terms of the memoir, I'm grateful for Bill Brody's early endorsement and the hours he spent working on his foreword and reviewing the manuscript. The NIH's John Burklow, a dedicated, whip-smart public servant, was another key supporter, providing a thorough review of an earlier draft of the manuscript, among other crucial help. It takes a village to achieve, and, accordingly, I have many more to thank for the creation of this book, including my brother, Moustafa, who provided countless hours of his time for interviews and the search for photos. Similarly, Mark Devlin was indispensable, aiding us in all stages of this book's creation and completion.

Other friends, colleagues, and family who reviewed all or part of the manuscript, provided invaluable insights, and/or allowed themselves to be interviewed, include Harold Varmus, Will Zerhouni, Adam Zerhouni, Ed Miller, Bob Carfagno, Marty Pomper, Marc Smolonsky, Amelia Arria, Keith Penn-Jones, Carey J. Kriz, Bill Drury, Suzie Holbrook, Armistead Williams, Gary Nabel, Phil Frost, Chris Viehbacher, Jeremy Berg, Lana Skirboll, David Bowen, Steven Rales, Ernesto Bertarelli, Sudip Parikh, Jim Greenwood, Mary Woolley, Michael Milken, Tony Fauci, Cheryl Jaeger, Elliot McVeigh, Ron Daniels, Richard Klausner, Thoms Insel, and the Office of George W. Bush. I'd also like to thank Christie Vera for all her efforts in supporting this project as well as Catherine Jacquet, who expertly coordinated much of the scheduling throughout this process.

In looking back on my life journey and the progressions of my career, there are many who I'd like to thank, including those mentioned in this book, for all they've contributed to my life and career. Nadia deserves the most praise of them all. She's the love of my life, my tireless supporter who has always believed in me. Without her, my American dream wouldn't have been possible.

I also want to recognize my earliest mentors who guided me immeasurably, including my parents, my uncle (Djillali Rahmouni), Stanley Siegelman, Bill Brody, and Bruce Holbrook as well as the many others who intersected with my life at various points. The rest of the names who deserve thanks could fill another book. Please know that even if you haven't been mentioned in this section, this memoir is a tribute to you. I couldn't have made it here without you. Thank you.

About the Author

Dr. Elias Zerhouni served as the fifteenth director of the National Institutes of Health (NIH) under President George W. Bush and as a presidential envoy for science and technology under President Barack Obama. He has worked as a global health research senior fellow at the Bill & Melinda Gates Foundation and served as president of research and development at Sanofi, a multinational pharmaceutical giant.

Zerhouni, who is Professor Emeritus Radiology and Biomedical Engineering at Johns Hopkins University, also served as chair of the Department of Radiology and executive vice dean of the School of Medicine. He is the author of more than 200 publications and an inventor whose research has saved countless patients with suspected lung or breast cancer from unnecessary surgeries and advanced the field of cardiovascular MRI. Zerhouni is president of OPKO Health, a multinational biopharmaceutical and diagnostics company, and cofounder of OPKO's ModeX Therapeutics, a biotechnology company focused on developing innovative, multispecific biologic drugs for cancer and infectious diseases. He is a board member for the Foundation for the National Institutes of Health, the Lasker Foundation, and Research!America. He is an elected member of the U.S. National Academy of Medicine and the U.S. National Academy of Engineering, and a recipient of the Legion of Honour medal from the French National Order.